PRACTICAL PLANNING IN MUSIC THERAPY FOR THE AGED

Ruth Bright, Mus. Bac. (Melbourne), C.M.T.
Music Therapist, Health Commission of
New South Wales, Australia

MAGNAMUSIC-BATON, INC.
10370 PAGE INDUSTRIAL BLVD.
ST. LOUIS, MO. 63132

Library of Congress Catalogue Number 81-84622

ISBN 0-941814-00-9

Published By Musicgraphics
124 Atlantic Ave., Lynbrook,
N.Y. 11563 U.S.A.
© 1981 Musicgraphics

TABLE OF CONTENTS

PREFACE
Definition of music therapy—examples of therapy programmes for all ages—aims of book.

P.1

INTRODUCTION
Outline of potential problems for the aged (physical, social, intellectual, emotional) as background of music therapy.

P.3

Chapter 1.
Music therapy and the physical needs of the frail aged. Need for mobility—combining individual work with counselling—music + physical therapy; exercise programme for wheel-chair patients (illustrated.)

P.7

Chapter 2.
The elderly patient in need of psychiatric care.
Variety of causes/diagnoses necessitating institutional care; suggested programmes for group work; benefits of various approaches. Special problems. Resource lists.

P. 16

Chapter 3.
Music in Rehabilitation.
Need for teamwork between all therapists; sensory losses and lateral neglect; group work for social contacts, intellectual stimulation. Programmes described, links with speech therapy discussed.

P. 27

Chapter 4.
Loss and grief in the aged.
Difficulties in loss and grief encountered by the aged; therapeutic intervention for the dying, bereaved, grieving; long-term therapy with the dying. Use of recorded music, and need for wide repertoire by therapist. Teamwork with other staff.

P. 33

Chapter 5.
Creativity in the aged through music therapy.
Value of learning new ideas and skills; use of instruments, improvisation.

P. 45

Summing-up.
Emphasis on music therapy as concerned with feelings rather than statistics, importance of self-esteem and communication as main function of music therapy in geriatrics.

P. 49

Photographs between pages 25 and 26.

PREFACE

What is music therapy? Many people reading those words will find that a carefully worded definition immediately comes to mind, such as:—

"Music therapy is the planned use of music to improve the functioning in his environment of an individual or a group of clients who have social, intellectual, physical or emotional needs of a special nature. Music therapy is carried out by a trained therapist working in the context of a clinical team."

The trouble with such a statement is that, unless you already know quite a lot, it does not really tell you very much about what music therapy is in practice; the uninformed listener tends to get a rather "glazed" look, and he usually goes on to say, "Yes, but what does a music therapist actually *do?*"

This is in some ways hard to explain, so diverse is the field of music therapy. The interested observer might see, for instance:—

- A therapist improvising atonal or pentatonic music on the piano or other instruments to help a client to express his hidden feelings, achieving a reflective approach in psychotherapy in individual or small group music-making.

- A group of patients lying on the floor, listening to recorded music while, to aid their relaxation, the music therapist describes a scene of tranquillity and beauty, which becomes the setting for imagined transactions between the patients and significant figures in their lives.

- A sing-along for elderly people in which each individual is able to choose his favourite song, and speaks about its significance in his life and relationships, or just joins in with others — or even merely listens.

- A group of young people listening to pop music and choosing cards with feelings written on them such as ANGER, PEACE, AGGRESSION, going on to talk about the appropriateness or otherwise of the choice of music/card for each person.

- A group of intellectually handicapped children singing about the colour of their T-shirts, or finding their ears and eyes, or miming the emergence of a butterfly from its cocoon, learning free movement and communication.

- An autistic child playing a chime bar, apparently lost in his own private world and yet relating through music to the therapist on the floor beside him.

1

- A group of psychiatric patients improvising music on tuned and untuned percussion instruments, investigating and revealing the relationships between the members of the group through their battles for musical cohesion, their subservience or leadership through melody and rhythm, all without a word being spoken.

- A brain-damaged car-accident victim learning to play the bongo drums, thereby improving hand-function and spatial awareness.

- A dying cancer patient re-building communication with his estranged wife by reminiscing about the music of their courtship days.

All these, and many many others, are instance of music therapy, but the casual observer might wonder what they had in common, and for some activities, such as group improvisation or singalongs, the untrained person might even wonder wherein lay the therapy. But the trained professional who is conversant with psychodynamics will see that below the surface of these different approaches lies not mere recreation but an awareness of the human need for communication and achievement and the building or re-building of positive relationships. He will see that, because of its impact on deep-seated feelings (feelings of which the client himself may be superficially unaware), music is an ideal medium for reaching those hidden emotions and for helping the individual to improve his functioning in the environment. And this basically is the same process, whether we are thinking of an intellectually handicapped child (low in self-esteem and in achievement), an elderly stroke patient, a young adult who is drug-dependent, or any other of the many types of clients with whom music therapists work.

This book to some extent is an answer to the question of the uninformed who ask "But what does a music therapist actually do?" It is also a "doing" book for those who are involved in music therapy but who feel that they need to improve their skills in work with the elderly, and who are seeking practical help in how to plan therapeutic programmes for the aged.

I am grateful to many people for help in preparing this book: — to my family for their patience and for practical help in proof-reading and indexing; to Dawn Wood for secretarial help and for doing the photography; to colleagues at Rozelle and Lidcombe Hospitals, Sydney; and most important of all, to my patients, who have taught me so much.

INTRODUCTION

In planning any therapeutic activity for the aged, it is necessary to have a clear understanding of their needs and the problems which they may encounter as life continues. By having such a clear understanding, we are the better able to plan our programmes and to make sure that they are truly therapeutic in aim. We can never be entirely certain of success, but at least we can *try!* It is in this detailed knowledge of the difficulties encountered by some of our aged population, the recognition of pathology when it occurs, the ability to work with other members of the clinical team and our ability to shape our music programmes to fit in with the total treatment plan that our music becomes therapy as distinct from recreation. In this there is (as with work with the intellectually handicapped, the physically disabled or the socially disadvantaged) a somewhat tenuous line between recreation or special education and therapy — there are many activities which, although intended as recreational or educational, do have a "therapeutic spin-off" (and this will be discussed in detail later — see pages 28, 29). But underlying a truly therapeutic programme there is always a plan (based on proper assessment and evaluation) and knowledge of the needs of the client, whether these are social, physical, intellectual or emotional.

What then are the special needs of the aged? It is common for those who work in the field of geriatrics to believe that almost every aged person needs care of some kind, that they will need either treatment for a physical ailment, help with depression or other mental illness, or will become so frail that they will need to be in an institution of some kind. But this is in fact not so: staff of hospitals and nursing homes are led to this tacit belief simply because the elderly people they meet are so in need, but in reality the majority of elderly people cope with life adequately, they continue to live independently to an advanced age, they manage their everyday living competently, and any diminution in physical capacity is far from being pathological. Some writers on aging have put the figure of those who need custodial care of some kind as low as 6%[1].

Despite this general level of health and independence, it is true nevertheless that we are today faced with a very large number of persons who need help of one variety or another. The explanation of this apparent paradox is that although the *percentage* of elderly people in need of care is small, the actual numbers are still high, simply because more people now reach old age. Those who are interested in such matters will find it helpful to read historical studies of life expectation and to see how the defeat (in general) of such childhood "killers" as measles and whooping cough, coupled with the general conquest of TB, has led to the large numbers of people who survive to old age [2]. Thus, despite the large numbers of elderly people living at home and enjoying their life-style, we are continually meeting people in hospitals and nursing homes who need a great deal of help of one kind or another.

Speaking at a congress on Gerontology in New Zealand in 1980, Professor John Brocklehurst, of the University of Manchester, U.K., spoke of the precarious balance maintained by the aged. He underlined the fact already mentioned, of the high percentage of elderly people who maintain good health and life style to the end of their lives, but spoke also of the fine edge on which such life-style is balanced, saying that it takes very little to destroy the equilibrium and create a situation of ill-health or social distress.

The factors involved in the equilibrium of living are those of physical well-being, social support, emotional stability and intellectual status. Before discussing the alteration to this balance which can be experienced by the aged, we need to consider first our own responses to difficulties. The young or middle-aged person can cope with a change of family structure fairly well, eventually adapting to loss of spouse, change of financial status and so on — not without sadness or stress, but in general, (depending on previous life-experiences and capacity to adapt), without complete collapse and without the necessity for admission to hospital. Similarly most people can cope with even serious illness or operation without loss of orientation and without loss of total intellectual capacity.

But with the aged this is frequently not so: a change which to a younger person would seem relatively trivial, such as a change of neighbours, can in the aged lead to utter social breakdown. A surgical operation which a younger person would "take in his stride" can, for the aged, lead to disorientation, apparent dementia, incontinence and other major sequellae. An illness such as pneumonia or a urinary tract infection, which has little or no impact on emotional stability or intellect for the young adult, can cause hallucinations and delusions in the aged, leading—if diagnosis is poor—to admission to a psychiatric unit. Relatives moving away, which would cause only sadness and a temporary sense of loss to a young person, can cause not only severe grief reactions in the aged but also — because of their need for social support both in practical and emotional terms — grave mental and physical deterioration. A minor defect such as corns on the feet, which a younger person would deal with adequately, can in the aged cause a frightening sequence of results, reminding one of the old story "for lack of a nail the battle was lost": uncomfortable feet cause wearing of sloppy slippers — unsteady walking — a fall — fractured femur — possible pneumonia if individual is lying on the floor for any length of time, or following surgery if post-operative ventilation is not maintained. Also possibility of decubitus ulcers ("pressure sores"), resulting usually not so much from poor nursing as from the prolonged period in which the unconscious patient is lying on the operating table with pressure on prominent areas such as the heels and the sacrum, and which pressure (by decreasing circulation) causes ulceration to develop shortly afterwards. An alternative "scenario" for the effects of corns on the feet is that, because walking is painful and slippers are worn, the individual tends to stay at home instead of going shopping, lives on an inadequate diet, and develops malnutrition with consequent generalized ill-health and mental deterioration.

Many such sequences can be described, all of which are genuine possibilities for the isolated elderly. These few examples will show clearly that the aged are very much "at risk" of things going wrong, that events which for a young person would be merely a nuisance, a disappointment or a challenge to adaptation are to the elderly a potential tragedy.

What has all this got to do with music therapy, and why does a music therapist need to know about either the statistics on illness in the aged or the possible appalling results of relatively minor problems?

Firstly, on the occurrence of illness and frailty in the aged: as has already been stated, it is common for those who are concerned in the care of the aged to assume that all aged people will suffer disability, mental deterioration or otherwise come to need custodial care of some kind. And this attitude or mistaken belief may make it hard for us to understand the patent resentment shown by those elderly people who do come into care. We may say, or merely think, "What is he grumbling about—doesn't he realize that this happens to all of us as we get older?" But the client/patient knows quite well that it does *not* happen to everyone, he probably knows many people of his own age who are still healthy and independent, and this adds to his frustration, his sadness, and even his bewilderment at being, as he may see it, singled out for misfortune. Unless we understand about these feelings, we are unlikely to be able to help him accept his residual disability—and since this area of counselling and help is very much the province of the music therapist, we must ensure that we are fully informed.

Secondly, this attitude, "But it happens to everyone!", can lead to inadequate medical care, and although this is not the precise area of work for the Music therapist, it needs to be mentioned. All too many medical practitioners still take the attitude that the aged must accept without question the inevitability of disease and disability, and that treatment should not be attempted past a certain age. The story told by Professor (now Sir) Ferguson Anderson, of Scotland, and quoted in various forms by several writers, illustrates well this attitude, and the response of at least one aged person to it. An elderly Scotsman went to his general practitioner about a painful knee; he was told, "Ah well, Angus, you are 94 now and you must expect that kind of thing!" To which Angus replied, "But my other knee is also 94 and it is NOT painful!" Angus was quite right in refusing to accept age itself as accounting for his difficulty, but many aged people are incapable of such a strong-minded response, and indeed their symptoms may by their very nature preclude such response, as with the apparent psychosis of the elderly lady admitted overnight to a Psychiatric Unit, who was found next morning to have a pneumonia which could (as the head of the Unit described it) "be heard across the room!" Unusual grief reactions may also confuse the picture, leading to a wrong diagnosis of psychosis or senile dementia, and although the music therapist would not often

5

challenge the diagnosis made by a senior medical officer, it is necessary for all of us to be aware of the possibility of wrong diagnosis and be ready tactfully to present our own observations on a patient's state of mind or other relevant information, especially if these seem to be in conflict with the pattern of behaviour observed by others.

Thus we can see that it is essential for music therapists to be no less well informed and educated than their colleagues from other disciplines, and although we may be concerned in very practical terms with planning music therapy activities for group or individual, activities designed to stimulate or maintain physical well-being, we should nevertheless be aware of the total pattern of life for each individual in our groups, so that we may adopt a wholistic approach to our therapy by inter-weaving music therapy with other modes of treatment and care.

This book is not intended to replace its forerunner, "Music in Geriatric Care" (re-issued in 1980), but to supplement it. Therapists are therefore advised to refer to this earlier book for discussion of specific diseases and conditions. Although topics are dealt with in different chapters, they are by no means mutually exclusive and therefore, if a particular subject is not discussed under what might appear to be its appropriate heading, it should appear elsewhere. Thus the use of percussion instruments is mentioned under "creativity", and so on. When doubtful, consult the index.

REFERENCES

1. Munnichs, J.M.A. and Bigot, A. *Psychology of Ageing, Long Term Illness and Death,* (in:—Textbook of Geriatric Medicine and Gerontology, ed. Brocklehurst, J., pub. Churchill Livingstone, Edinburgh and London, 1973).
2. Pressat, R., *Population,* pub. Watts, London (The New Thinker's Library), 1970.

RECOMMENDED READING

Comfort, A. *A Good Age,* pub. Beazley, U.K., 1977 (different editions, giving approprate resource lists for various countries - title remains unaltered).
Hawker, M. *Geriatrics for Physiotherapists and the Allied Health Professions,* pub. Faber & Faber, London, 1974.
Burnside, I.M. (Editor). *Nursing and the Aged,* pub. McGraw-Hill, 1981.
Exton-Smith, A.N. (Editor). *Care of the Elderly,* pub. New York Academic Press, Gruna & Stratton, New York, 1977.
Bright, Ruth. *Music in Geriatric Care,* re-issued Musigraphics, N.Y., U.S.A. 1980.

CHAPTER 1: MUSIC THERAPY AND THE PHYSICAL NEEDS OF THE FRAIL AGED

In order to enjoy our old age, it is necessary to remain as fit as possible so that we are not prevented from following our ordinary social life or our chosen hobbies merely because our bodies let us down. In physical fitness, there is a "luck factor" involved, presumably of genetic origin or resulting from health/illness earlier in life, so that some people simply cannot remain fit no matter how hard they try and no matter how carefully they watch their weight, drinking habits, etc. But even given a degree of physical disability such as osteoarthritis, some loss of hearing or sight or other problem, we would hope still to be able to enjoy living and still be able to take our place in society. To be involved in a fitness programme designed for our appropriate age is wise — a check-up with one's medical adviser would be a sensible precaution, but, with his approval, it can only do good to take part in sport or a keep-fit group of some kind.

But what of those who have suffered a disease or accident which precludes such involvement? For many such people, physiotherapy (physical therapy) will be prescribed for specific treatment of specific disorders, and, although teamwork for such therapy is not common, those who do adopt a team approach find it so helpful to the patient that in time to come it may be accepted standard procedure. At the Caulfield Rehabilitation Hospital in Melbourne, the physiotherapists (as physical therapists are called in Australia) work with the music therapist in preparing cassettes of music which is helpful to the programmes of exercises to be followed by stroke and other patients. These are changed regularly so that the patient does not lose interest in the idea, but always the music selected is such as to enhance the performance of exercises in the actual movements performed, and also makes the activity more enjoyable so that the patient is more conscientious and persistent in carrying the exercises out each day. In the Department at the Hospital, ear-phones are used so that people in different cubicles or areas of the therapy gymnasium are not disturbed, and then, when the patient is discharged home on an Out Patient basis, returning to the Hospital for day treatment and maintenance as long as is necessary, the cassettes are used at home with or without earphones.

Music has several functions in the carrying out of physiotherapy exercises, one of which is seen in the programme described above, i.e. the enhancement of enjoyment and therefore of persistence. But this is not the only function — music also appears to affect the pain threshold for some people: it is recognized that there are psychological/emotional components to the perception of pain and it may be therefore that, for an anxious person, music helps to alleviate anxiety and thus lessens the perception of severity of pain.

The observations which have led to the formulation of this as-yet untested hypothesis have been concerned with post-operative orthopaedic patients, people who are weight-bearing for the first time after repair of fractured femur, or who are in the early stages of ambulation following this or similar surgical procedures. Patients who are in traction or who are temporarily on bed-rest also benefit from music therapy at the bedside, because the rhythm of the music assists them in moving the affected limb (even if only to "wiggle" the toes — and this, small a movement though it is, is helpful in maintaining circulation and thus, in theory at any rate, assisting the healing processes).

In planning this use of music in therapy, the essentials to bear in mind are:—

1. The physical therapist must be happy at such co-operative work.
2. The music must be played personally rather than on a record, so that the speed can be adjusted at will to match the speed of movement of the patient at any time.
3. The patient must him/herself enjoy music so that the activity is seen as adding "fun" to the proceeding.
4. The music selected should ideally be familiar to the patient so that he can sing the tune if he wishes, or at least recognize it, and of course it must be a tune which is liked by the patient — a tune which one hated could hardly be helpful!

The actual tune selected will depend on the age and cultural background of the patient as well as on the type of movement which is to be attempted. The tune "Ain't she sweet, see her coming down the street" has proved successful on a number of occasions in the author's experience, partly because the rhythm and the general jaunty atmosphere of the song suit the activity, but also because the words themselves are to some extent appropriate to the occasion — walking down a hospital corridor, leaning on a walking frame and supported by therapists or nurses, can not truly be called "sweet" and yet there is sufficient truth to give everyone a cheerful feeling — if someone has been unable to walk for a long time and has had a total hip replacement or has had a femur repaired, a knee re-modelled or some other orthopaedic procedure carried out to improve mobility, everyone can share in the patient's satisfaction that soon she *will* be walking down the street again!

For persons who have had an amputation, that particular song is perhaps too jolly, and a quiet waltz might be more appropriate — although this decision would depend on the attitude and outlook of the patient. (A waltz may seem inappropriate rhythmically, but if played at the correct tempo, used with one bar for each step, a waltz makes good walking music. It must be played in strict time, without any hint of rubato, to avoid confusion and loss of rhythm in the movement.)

Stroke patients, amputees and others are often given pulley work to be done, i.e. apparatus is set up in which the patient has a hand-grip on which to pull, and weights are attached to the end of the rope over the pulley, or springs are used, which help to build up arm muscles. Whilst this is essential for certain conditions, it is nonetheless a very boring activity, and here recorded music chosen by the patient can be used, or personally-presented music can be played if time permits, so that the music is added to personal conversation. Such one-to-one opportunity for therapeutic dialogue may be valuable for those patients who are having difficulty adjusting to their acquired disability. The author has clear memories of one such conversation with an amputee about the difficulties he was having with sexual intercourse because of a problem which had developed in his stump some months after the original surgery. This aspect of amputation is often not dealt with adequately (although it is perhaps wrong to single out the rehabilitation of amputees for this criticism — all too often the attitude taken in rehabilitation in general is "You are lucky to be alive, so why worry about sex?" But it is still true that, whilst most people are aware that strokes, spinal injuries, spasticity, etc., cause severe difficulties in sexual relationships, we do not always recognize the problems of the male above-knee amputee.) It is unlikely that the music therapist will be able to offer any immediate solutions to the problems which are revealed in such one-to-one conversations, whether they are concerned with marital relationships or any other aspects of living. What the music therapist can do is to bring these problems to the attention of other members of staff who are able to offer help or appropriate advice. The other benefit of such intimate dialogue is that merely to talk about the problem may be part-way to solving it, so long as one's response to the presentation of worries is not to brush them aside and say "Don't worry — you'll be all right!" Nothing is more frustrating and irritating than to find that, having been desperate enough to talk about a deep-seated anxiety or fear, this fear is then dealt with superficially. Even if all the patient wants is to be reassured that his fears are groundless, this reassurance must be given seriously, not with laughing half-contempt. If the fear is concerned with something outside our own area of work, then we must respond by saying "I really don't know about that, but would you like me to ask the doctor/social worker/physio to talk to you about it?" This response must be the same whether a patient is trying to find out how soon his cancer is to be fatal, when he will get his artificial limb, whether his cataract operation has been successful, or why his tablets for his "heart condition" are different from those of his next-door neighbour at home.

In this, as in so many aspects of music therapy, it is hard to differentiate clearly between music for physical problems and music for emotional problems; it demonstrates vividly the balance which the therapist must maintain between the musical side of the work and the therapeutic/medical side. (See also p. 27, 39).

In the hospital, many patients will be having formal physical therapy and will therefore not require general keep-fit work or what is often called Maintenance Therapy. However in nursing homes and in psychiatric hospitals, where concentrated physical therapy is not given, or for those hospital patients who are not receiving physical therapy as part of their prescribed treatment, the music therapist is likely to be involved in exercise programmes. Clearance must be obtained from a doctor for any frail or ill patient before starting on a programme of exercises, but for the majority of psychiatric elderly patients and for many nursing home patients, the nursing staff will be able to assess the suitability of any individual for inclusion in group exercises.

The programme here described was devised by Ms Hartley-Smith of the Health Commission of New South Wales, Australia, as being suitable for wheelchair patients in general, and some of the exercises were intended to be especially helpful to hemiplegic stroke patients. I am grateful to Ms Hartley-Smith for permission to include the programme here, and to Ms Diana Rankin for permission to include the sketches she drew for a meeting of the Australian Music Therapy Association, when the exercise programme was presented as part of a workshop in geriatrics.

WHEELCHAIR EXERCISES

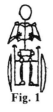

Fig. 1

1. Fingers on lower ribs in front, breathing in through the nose and out through the mouth. Three times *only*. Use simple sequence of slow chords.

Fig. 2

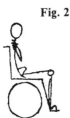 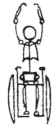 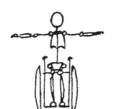 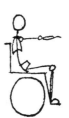 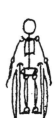

2. Raise both arms from starting position with hands on the shoulders to reach upwards — sideways — forwards — downwards, coming back to shoulder between each change. 4 times cycle. For hemiplegic patient, assist affected arm with "good" arm.

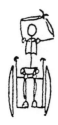

Accompaniment — any slow, waltz, such as Skaters' Waltz etc.

3. Before starting, lift up foot-plate of wheelchair. Raise knees and feet, then lower, "marching" on the spot. Eight times is recommended for frail patients.

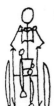 **Fig. 3**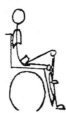

Hemiplegics may lean across to assist affected leg. Any brisk march is suitable, or the song "Knees up Mother Brown."

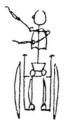 **Fig. 4**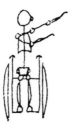

4. Turn the trunk from side to side, letting arms swing loosely. 6 times. Slow waltz is suitable as accompaniment.

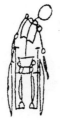 **Fig. 5**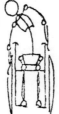

5. Bending down sideways, alternately, letting the arms hang loosely. 6 times. Similar music to exercise 4.

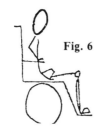

Fig. 6

6. Hands on sides of chair, push body up while tightening the buttocks at the same time. This exercise assists arm strength but also strengthens muscles of the pelvic floor, thereby helping to prevent incontinence. Waltz tempo is suitable. Do 6 times.

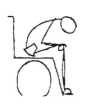

Fig. 7

7. Lean forwards slightly, head towards knees, hands on knees. Then straighten up and arch back, but with head up, chin tucked in. Waltz tempo. 6 times.

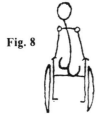

Fig. 8

8. Hands on sides of chair, roll from one buttock to the other. 6 times. The "Skye Boat Song" is helpful for this exercise. (The sketch shows the back view of the patient as he/she sits in the wheelchair.)

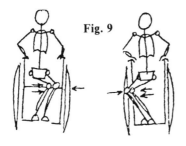

Fig. 9

9. Feet on *floor*, knees together: swing knees from side to side, resist the movement with the other knee or hand to build strength. 8 times. The Scots tune "Keel Row" (slowly) will be suitable.

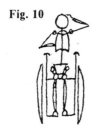

Fig. 10

10. Place one hand behind the neck and the other in the middle of the back. Change the position of the hands alternately; this gives a complete range of movement for the shoulder. A hemiplegic person will only do this with the unaffected arm, but if the affected shoulder is pain-free, the other arm can be moved passively by the therapist. Suitable music is a march, some patients may require a complete bar of music to do the changeover movement.

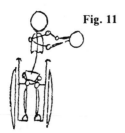 **Fig. 11**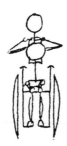

11. Ball throwing in pairs can be included in the exercise programme when patients are not severly disabled. Throw centrally and then to either side. Waltz music may be used to accompany this action, but it may not be possible for everyone to keep the precise rhythm going.

This programme of exercises is suitable for wheelchair patients and also for psychogeriatric groups. Extension of the head and neck must be avoided, as also must movements which involve leaning forward more than a few inches. If recorded music is used, it may be necessary for the therapist to set the music going and go round to assist with various movements. Patients should be instructed to stop the exercise after the appropriate number of repetitions in order to avoid fatigue before the programme is complete.

The session should end with diaphragmatic breathing, hands on ribs as in exercise 1, and it will also be helpful to repeat breathing exercise between 4-8 in order to maintain adequate oxygen for the working muscles and also to give the client a chance to relax briefly. But in each "breather" only do 3 breaths to avoid the possibility of hyperoxygenation and consequent dizziness.

Music suitable for various types of movements:

1. *Brisk, firm and fairly rapid movement:* Marches of any kind, played by brass band or Scottish pipe bands. The latter must be selected with care in case the pipes are disliked by the patient or in case the music itself is of very mournful atmosphere. Scottish country dances are also suitable, e.g. "The Dashing White Sergeant", any music written for The Lancers, etc.

2. *Slower, gentler movements, or slow walking:* Any waltz tunes if played and planned for dancing, not for listening, (e.g. many Strauss waltzes are suitable only if played in strict tempo, since when played as "concert" items, the speed varies too often for use in exercise programme).

   Some more modern music can be used if beat is regular, e.g. Beatles' "When I'm 64". Although this is in itself a brisk melody, the "beat" is such that it can be used for quite slow movements. Many elderly people also enjoy Rock and Roll music from the 1950's, e.g. "Rock Around the Clock", recorded by Bill Haley and The Comets.

3. *Music of 'Foreign' origin.* In countries such as Australia where there is a large number of new migrants who still speak only their original tongue, there is a need for sound knowledge of music from the countries from which the people have come. Thus a Polish Mazurka may be (and has been shown to be) of inestimable value to a non-English speaking migrant, who has been helped to feel at home with certain physio procedures through the use of the music, played personally on the accordion. But in the U.S.A., where the era of new migration is in general over, so that most people with "foreign" names have in fact been born in U.S.A. and are able to speak English, the need for ethnic music is less urgent. But it may prove helpful with some individuals to be able to play music from their ancestral country in times of special need or loneliness. The Italian melody, "Tirritomba", is one such rhythmic tune, the melody "In Ushkadara"* has, in the author's experience, helped people from a variety of countries, since it is known — at varying speeds — to people from Greece, Turkey, Yugoslavia, Russia, Crete and Arabic countries. By using ethnic music, we may be able to assist the physical therapy programme to be carried out more effectively, even with people who have become fairly well assimilated into their country of choice.

Music therapy does combine well with physical approaches in treatment, and, because the benefits are clearly visible to therapists from other professions, involvement with physical therapy does bring to the music therapist an immediate recognition and appreciation which does not always occur when emotional needs are dealt with. Nevertheless it seems wrong for music therapists to concentrate overmuch on integrating music therapy with physical therapy, except where there are special needs — as,

* From "Music Sounds Afar" — see Resource List, Chapter 2.

for instance, in the mobilizing of the withdrawn psychiatric patient, or overcoming fear and anxiety in the post-operative patient. In his book, "The Elderly Australian"[1], Dr. Bruce Ford has written briefly about all the professions involved in rehabilitation and care of the elderly. Writing about music therapists, he has said that there are already too many people concentrating on elderly people's gut and bones, and not enough working with their feelings. Dr. Ford suggests that it is more valuable for music therapists to help the aged with their emotional needs, their need to cry or laugh, than to help with their exercises. Although this was written about life "Down Under," it is probably true also of life "On Top," and it is the opinion of the author that — despite all the attractions of working in an area which tends to bring instant recognition from the other professions — we ought to spend our major efforts on the emotional and psychological needs of the aged, integrating this with physical activities only when there are some special needs in motivation or the like.

When we are working in a programme which concerns the physical needs of the aged sick, we must always have in the back of our minds the emotional problems which are experienced by our patients in coping with their disabilities, so that we can use music to help these, even if we appear at that moment to be dealing only with the body.

REFERENCES

1. Ford, Bruce. *The Elderly Australian,* p.113, pub. Penguin (paperback), Ringwood, Australia, 1976.

CHAPTER 2: THE ELDERLY PATIENT IN NEED OF PSYCHIATRIC CARE

In today's publications we are faced with a bewildering variety of terms to describe elderly people in need of psychiatric care — we read of psychogeriatrics, of geronto-psychiatry, of the psychiatry of the elderly, and so on. However, for the purposes of this book, no philosophy of nomenclature will be adopted, and terms will be used as they happen to be convenient.

In the institutions which used to be called Mental Hospitals and before that, Asylums, there are many and varied reasons for people being placed therein. In many ways it seems a pity that the word Asylum has become a dirty word — it used to have connotations of protection and refuge, a sense in which it is still used when we speak of political refugees seeking asylum from their enemies. And surely there is even today a sense in which psychiatric hospitals provide this refuge for some people from a world with which they cannot cope. The current trend towards discharge into the community is regarded by many as mere faddism which takes little account of the real needs of the people thus discharged and in many cases means merely that they exchange one institution (the psychiatric hospital) for another (the hostel or boarding house).[1,2] And because such places are often not suited to a person who has for a long time lived in the protected environment of a psychiatric hospital, there are re-admissions when such people are unable to cope with ordinary community living, or when hostels/nursing homes, etc., are unable to cope with their behaviour — disinhibition, incontinence, changes to day/night living patterns and so on. As well as re-admissions of this kind, there have always been people whose mental state followed a cyclical pattern, necessitating periodic admission.

The significance to the music therapist of this pattern of discharge/re-admission is that one is likely to meet the same people over and over again, and it is essential that such people should be able to join in music therapy sessions, since music has been observed by the writer, over the last 21 years, to offer greater sense of security and continuity than almost any other activity.

This sense of security is not, of course, confined to the aged — a youngster suffering from leukemia told the charge sister of a children's ward that she did not dread coming back into hospital quite so much because she knew that each week there would be music and she could play her recorder and have some fun.

One matter of which music therapists need to be aware in planning programmes is the tremendous variety of diagnoses which may be met in a unit for the elderly psychiatric patient, or in an institution set aside for elderly people whose mental state makes custodial care necessary. In one unit/ward we may see: —

- Post-cerebro-vascular accident (stroke) cases who have suffered a change in personality or whose intellect has been sufficiently impaired to make independent life impossible, or who have become socially disinhibited, thereby losing the normal restraints of behaviour which are necessary for family-living.

- Post-motor vehicle accident or brain surgery cases, who have similar problems.

- Patients with late-onset schizophrenia or other psychosis, or with continuing psychoses from earlier life.

- "Burnt-out" psychoses — people whose primary psychiatric illness has ceased to have any florid existence, but who have become so dependent and/or disinhibited over the years that it is only possible for them to live in a psychiatric institution.

- Patients suffering from Korsakow's syndrome, whose alcohol abuse has caused this particular combination of mental and physical disabilities, which render ordinary community life impossible.

- People who have, as the result of arterio-sclerosis, Alzheimer's Disease, or other deterioration of neurones, suffered such memory loss as to make independent life impossible, and whose behaviour makes it difficult/impossible for hostels or the like to tolerate their behaviour.

- Those people whose Parkinson's disease has caused mental disturbance to the extent that custodial care is needed.

- Persons with Huntington's Disease, in whom the psychiatric symptoms are severe. (Many Huntington's Disease patients are cared for in ordinary nursing homes because their physical disability is such that behaviour problems are thereby reduced. But this is not so for all — some people retain sufficient physical power as to be able to cause grave problems with aggression and thus make life in a nursing home unavailable to them.)

- Elderly persons with severe intellectual handicap — persons who in past generations have usually succumbed to respiratory or other illnesses in their middle years but who now, thanks to antibiotics, etc., survive to middle and old age. Some such people have been in institutions all their lives, others have had to be admitted to institutional care when their parents have died or become so elderly and frail as to make it impossible for them to care for their retarded "children."

- People who have a combination of diseases — thus one meets people who have multiple sclerosis as well as some psychiatric illness (some may even have developed a psychiatric illness as a consequence of the M.S.). As well as conditions which may have a psychiatric component in themselves, we meet people in whom psychiatric illness and physical disease appear to co-exist without any causal relationship, and in all such cases we must be aware of their special needs as modified by both physical and psychiatric illness.

- Those with depressive states so severe that institutional care is needed.

In situations in which a group session makes it unlikely that the therapist will routinely be informed of all diagnoses, the music therapist must be able to "spot" cases which present an unusual picture and check on diagnosis, following this up by reading appropriate textbooks and asking advice from nursing staff/medical staff in order to understand the particular needs and limitations which are symptomatic of the disease. For instance, a patient who has had a bulbar palsy (from a lesion of the brain-stem) will usually (as well as suffering from varying degrees of paralysis, depending on the extent of the lesion) be found to be tearful and easily aroused emotionally, so that music may evoke apparent sadness. But many such persons are not in fact feeling sad at all, the tears are simply part of an emotional lability, they enjoy even the music which makes them cry, and to be excluded from the music session because it *appears* to make them unhappy, would be anti-therapeutic. This is but one instance of the approach needed by a music therapist, to understand the total picture of disease and disability presented by the members of the group or by individuals who are seen singly.

How then do we plan a programme for the psychogeriatric group? Usually the elderly patient benefits from group work since it promotes social interaction, and awareness of the world outside.

Many themes can be used: it is a mistake to have too many ideas in one session, or to use the same theme too often, but some repetition is helpful as giving comfortable familiarity.

Suggested Programme (To last not more than 40-45 minutes)

Prepare a box with objects which suggest songs — a Teddy bear, a scented rose, and old straw hat, a small brown jug, etc., etc., depending on cultural background and ethnic origin of group. Set up group (preferably 12-15, or less) in circle.

1. Session starts with welcome song — made up by the therapist and used each week in the same way (e.g. to tune "Good morning, we've danced the whole night through" — "Good morning, Mrs...., it's nice to see you here, good morning, good morning to you.")

2. Discuss weather, ask if anyone has noticed whether it is rainy or sunny. Sing appropriate song, as suggested by patients — or therapist, if no ideas from group.

3. Put objects on floor in centre of circle. Ask for suggestions for songs these objects remind them of. Pass rose around, ask whether anyone called Rose, or whether someone in their family of that name. Sing, e.g., "Sweet Rosie O'Grady," "Roses of Picardy," "Yellow Rose of Texas" — ask if rose which was passed around is correct colour or not. "Red Roses for a Blue Lady," etc., as requested.

4. After about ten minutes, play a march and ask people to stamp/tap feet on the floor, seated or standing depending on physical health.

5. Completing title of, say, three songs: "It's a long way to...... (Tipperary)," "The Atchison, Topeka and the......(Santa Fe)," etc.

6. Clapping to music — alter speed of music (faster-slower), see whether group can detect and respond to changes in tempo.

7. Return to cue objects, play "Old Straw Hat" — pass round copy of songsheet if possible. Ask whether anyone remembers who sang it? (Shirley Temple) What was the film? When did it come out? Did anyone see it? Where? Who did they go with? etc., etc. — stimulate as much reminiscence as possible. About 3-5 minutes perhaps.

8. Join hands around circle and play slow waltz, people move hands, sway to and fro. (Stimulates sense of belonging in the group, creates some measure of social bonding.)

9. End with "Auld Lang Syne" or similar End of Programme song which is familiar to group. Or therapist makes one up and uses it consistently each week.

Small segments of this can be used for severely deteriorated and demented patients on an individual basis or in groups of 2/3/4, encouraging reminiscence and awareness of therapist before introducing group concept.

Similar programmes can be used with variations, e.g. a sketch instead of objects; a newspaper session + songs from countries mentioned in the news + map of the world; seasons of the year with emphasis on gardening and farming + songs to suit.

In planning the objects to be brought, one must assess the general background to ensure that the members of the group do not experience undue failure. People of British origin will associate oranges and lemons with the song of that name (which is about the bell "tunes" of various ancient London churches, such as St. Clement's, St. Martin's and so on), but people without this prior knowledge will not know the song. Other people may know "The Teddy Bears' Picnic," and recall that tune on seeing a Teddy Bear — it is interesting to see the "cuddling response" which many elderly psychiatric, or other, patients show when the Teddy is passed around the circle. Perhaps this indicates a profound need for something to love, a need which is seldom met for such patients.

The advantages of using an object to stimulate choice of songs are several:

- it causes the people in the group to think (which is not so likely if the group leader just chooses the song and announces it);
- it gives extra stimuli and sensory in-put — one feels the texture of the bear's fur, one sniffs the tang of orange or lemon, one hears the tinkle of the sleigh bells as they are passed around;
- it provides a sense of decision-making for the members of the group. The therapist will have planned what songs are likely to be suggested by the objects brought, but to each patient there is a challenge and a decision — and in fact it does happen that one object will evoke memories of more than one song, some of which may be unknown to the therapist.

Similar advantages follow from using a sketch. Ideally this should be done on the spot by the therapist, on a large sheet of card or paper, or on a blackboard/whiteboard. Do not worry in case your drawing is pretty comical — it may even be very good for the patient's morale if it is bad — they then have the delightful feeling, (or some of them may), "I could do better than *that!*" All too often the staff in a hospital for the elderly must appear omnipotent — we can walk, we can talk, we can make decisions about our own lives, and above all we can go home at the end of the day. Thus to see a member of staff doing a perfectly terrible drawing on a blackboard can be of tremendous value to the patient. Pictures can be, and in fact should be, simple: it is sometimes helpful to build them up gradually, starting off for instance with a tree.

Songs which this may suggest could include: —

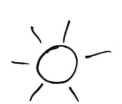

"Don't sit under the apple tree,"

"In the shade of the old apple tree,"

"Underneath the spreading chestnut tree,"

"I think that I shall never see, a poem lovely as a tree," (To which some may add the Ogden Nash couplet, "In fact unless the billboards fall, I'll never see a tree at all!")

Next add a stereotyped sketch of the sun: —

"You are my sunshine,"

"My old Kentucky home,"

"The sunshine of your smile."

Shade in some blue for the sky: —

"Blue Skies" (the Bing Crosby favourite).

Add a few birds: —

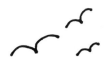

"Blue birds over the White Cliffs of Dover,"

"The bluebird of happiness,"

"Birdsong at eventide."

This building-up process can be continued until interest palls, or until the therapist's imagination runs out.

Passing round a rose can be extraordinarily productive — it has a pleasant scent (assuming that one has chosen a scented variety!), it reminds people of many special occasions in life as well as the pleasure of gardening, and it reminds one of many songs about roses, real or metaphorical. ("Roses of Picardy," "The Rose of No Man's Land," "My Wild Irish Rose," "Sweet Rosie O'Grady," "The Yellow Rose of Texas," etc., etc.)

Sample Programme No. 2:

Use a quiz format, e.g. working through the alphabet, asking people to suggest songs starting with the letter A,B,C, etc. For some people this may not be possible, but it has proved surprisingly successful with many patients who had been thought to be too out of touch with reality to cope with such a demanding session. The songs which people will know will depend on their family, culture and place of living, and if a tune is requested which the therapist does not know, the person asking for it may be invited to sing it for the group while it is recorded for future occasions — this is helpful for self-esteem as well as helpful to the therapist's repertoire. One severely deteriorated patient surprised the writer when, on reaching the letter "J" without anyone being able to suggest a song, the title of "O Johnny" was mentioned — Mr. B. said "But that's cheating, it starts with O not J!" One could use songs from each State as another basis.

When following a quiz pattern, whether it is songs from different countries of the world (using a map or globe to add interest to the programme), or any other basis, be ready to interpose different items in case of boredom, by playing records or tapes which fit in with the general theme, having some mobilization work, showing pictures of instruments from a particular country or interesting artefacts.

One can, for instance, take a particular country such as Ireland or Britain, show large travel posters of well-known places, play music from that country, pass around interesting items made there and so on; in this programme the quiz aspect would be of minor importance, but to use even a few questions does help to maintain alertness.

The techniques described here for building a group programme for re-orientation and discussion are also suitable for a group in geriatric rehabilitation or long-stay care, but in a psychogeriatric group can usually not be so fully developed in the way of discussion or further implications for the songs chosen. (see Chapter 3).

Recorded music — is there a place for it? It is acceptable to use recorded music if, for example, one is taking a mobilization group working alone; it is possible to stimulate movement and general participation on one's own whilst playing an instrument, if it is portable (e.g. accordion), but it is not easy. It may be more effective to put on a record or a tape and go around giving personal encouragement and help. But for sing-alongs or free choice sessions, there is no place for recorded music. Music must be played by a live performer/accompanist, who can transpose music up or down as needed, modified by the pitch of the voices. (Many songbooks are written in keys which are too high for the ordinary person to sing with comfort, and this alone accounts for much non-participation by members of a group.)

Some patients in a psychogeriatric group can and do enjoy listening to music by "serious" composers, and will enjoy a brief segment in the programme on the Composer of the Week. But for such work it is necessary to be selective, since the deterioration commonly found amongst such groups makes it probable that the activity will succeed with only small numbers. This type of work appears to be more successful in a geriatric rehabilitation group generally; nevertheless, one should not assume unquestioningly that it is pointless to "try" serious music; even amongst the most gravely ill or the most severely deteriorated people, one finds from time to time an individual whose life-history and experiences make the use of such music both enjoyable and necessary. One may postulate, for instance, a former opera singer or Lieder singer for whom the playing of "his" type of music would achieve more effective communication than the playing of "Daisy Bell" or "Frankie and Johnny."

Familiarity with music from many different places throughout the world is also helpful, so that memories of family music-making may be reached when working with people who are of migrant origin, even if the actual migration took place some time ago.

Special Problems:

Probably the most acute problems in work with the mentally disturbed elderly person are those of anger, aggression and intolerance, which — together with severe memory loss — challenge the music therapist (and indeed every other therapist) to every ounce of tact and ingenuity in his make-up. What do you do if a forgetful patient asks for a song to be played as soon as she has drawn breath from singing this song, simply because she has forgotten that it has just been played? And what do you do when other members of the group, intolerant of such forgetfulness (perhaps because of fear of their own similar eventual deterioration), react to the request by saying angrily, "But we've just *had* that!!" What do you do when two patients shape up for a fist-fight because they disagree on what song should be sung next? And what do you do when a wandering patient in his endlesss walking around the room bumps into another patient in the group, and gets a push which lands him on the floor?

Without wishing to paint too grim a picture of life in a ward for disturbed and deteriorated elderly people, these are the sort of incidents which tend to punctuate a music therapy session, and it would be unrealistic to suggest otherwise — the therapist must have some strategies with which to cope in such problems.

As with very young children, one needs to develop techniques of distraction so that the person who continually asks for the same song, because of memory loss, is met by a reply such as "That's a good idea — we'll have it soon, after we've sung Mr. Buckley's request and a few others". The same memory loss which causes the repetition of the request will prevent the person from remembering the reply, so that the second performance can be delayed for a while — but it should eventually be played again to keep faith with the individual's request.

One can also use distraction techniques when a fight is in the offing, using whatever suggestion seems most likely to succeed, e.g. "Do either of you know that song, 'On Top of Old Smokey'?," or some equally well-known song (but not the one which is the subject of the argument at that time), and then start playing it immediately. This does not always work, but it often does.

It is the demanding patient with a loud voice who probably poses the most difficult problem — the writer has one such person in a regular group, and his method is to sing *extremely* loudly — and accurately — the song he wants, with no regard at all for the request of anyone else. This would be not so bad if everyone in the group was happy to join in with his ideas, but other patients become upset/angry/tearful because their ideas are not getting a turn. We have tried ignoring him and singing the other songs requested, while he sings his songs, but the sheer volume of sound from Mr. G. spoils the pleasure of this; we have tried *asking* him to be quiet — he responds with a flow of obscenity and violent speech, together with threats of bodily aggression. We have tried asking nurses to remove him from the group — this results in actual violence followed later by lurid tales of unwarranted attacks by staff, etc., etc. The answer seems to be a compromise, in which Mr. G. is encouraged to choose a few songs, tolerance of other patients is requested in a way which flatters their own behaviour, and eventually Mr. G. settles down. But this type of behaviour is not easy to manage and demands great self-control from the therapist, and also considerable self-esteem since it can be damaging to be subjected to language which is vitriolic as well as obscene, and to threats of physical attack.

Some difficult patients can be managed by giving them a role in the group — asking them to hand out songbooks, find the place for those who do not see well, and in other ways boosting their self-esteem. But there is no one easy answer to any of these difficult situations.

In some areas one feels that patients fit into two broad categories — those who refuse to move at all willingly and those who never stop moving! Whilst it is not usually difficult to achieve some contact (however fleeting) with the immobile, the restless patient presents problems in communication. For the demented wanderer, who walks to and fro all day, the ability of the therapist to play a portable instrument is vital since it may give the opportunity for making at least a temporary relationship through music. Whilst the picture this conjures up to the inexperienced, (of the therapist trying to keep up with a wandering patient, playing/singing as she goes), may seem merely comical, those who are familiar with the difficulties of coping with such patients will know that even a peripatetic contact is valuable!

Choice of Material:

The ideal songbook for work in geriatrics, whether in psychogeriatrics or geriatric rehabilitation —

(a) is printed in large print,

(b) contains songs of the appropriate "vintage",

(c) is easily handled by the frail,

(d) has an accompaniment written in appropriate keys for the aged voice, unless the therapist is sufficiently good at transposition as to be able to do it at sight — which of course one *should* be, but we all have differing gifts in therapy!

The only song book known to the author which fulfils these parameters is that published during April, 1981, by Ulverscroft Large Print Books, their Large Print Songbook with music. (The words-only edition has been available for some ten years.) The music for this book was collated by a member of the Australian Music Therapy Association, who is not herself a therapist, but who has interests in the care of the aged. Accompaniments were planned for elderly people themselves rather than for music therapists, so the chords are simple and the notes are in large print, but therapists will find it a helpful source of old songs. To some extent it is influenced by its Australian/British origin, so that the American therapist will need to supplement it with songs native to the U.S.A. Some volumes of Folk Songs will be helpful (see list below) and a book of songs for each state of the Union will also be useful (see below also).

Whatever materials are used to add to the liveliness of a session, the aim should remain the same —

• to gain maximum participation from those who are usually uninvolved with living,

- to sing songs about the weather which will help them look outside the walls of the ward or hospital,
- to listen to music from countries which are "in the news" to add interest to a newspaper group,
- to add music from different eras in their personal lives to encourage reminiscence and the life review,
- to choose songs which mention colours to help each person be aware of his neighbour, even if at first that awareness is confined to looking at the colour of his or her clothes,
- to sing songs which mention people's names for the same aim of social interaction.

By doing this we will certainly gain some interaction, and even if this proves to be only short-lived, it is still worth doing. Even temporary miracles are worthwhile!

REFERENCES

1. Parker, Gordon. *Discharged Long-stay Psychiatric Patients,* pub. Health Commission of N.S.W., Sydney, Australia, 1974.
2. Braceland, F.J., *Editorial,* pp.15ff. in Yearbook of Psychiatry and Applied Mental Health, 1975, Braceland, F.J. et al editors, pub. Yearbook Medical Publishers, Chicago, U.S.A., 1975.

SUGGESTED READING

Aging and Mental Health, Butler, R.N. & Lewis, M.I., pub. C.V. Mosby & Co., St. Louis, U.S.A., 1973.
Nursing and the Aged, edited Burnside, pub. McGraw-Hill, 1981. Especially chapter on Reality Therapy, by D.R. Scarbrough, p.200ff.

RESOURCE BOOKS

Belafonte, H. *Songs Belafonte Sings,* pub. Duell, Sloan & Pearce, New York, U.S.A., 1962.
Charters, A. (Ed.), *Ragtime Songbook,* pub. Oak, New York, 1965.
Dunson, J. (Ed.), *Anthology of American Folk Music,* pub. Oak, New York, 1973.
Edwards, R. *The Big Book of Australian Folk Songs,* pub. Rigby, Adelaide, Australia, 1976.

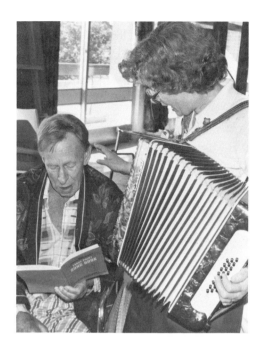

This patient is able to read the words of the song and enjoys singing despite his aphasia which has resulted from a lesion to the dominant hemisphere.

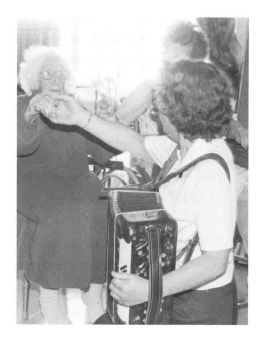

The therapist must be able to play from floor level in order to gain eye-contact with some frail patients.

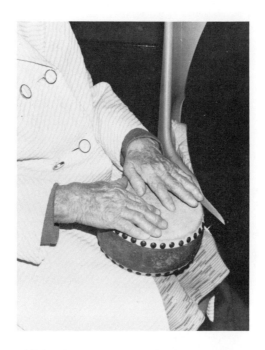

Using instruments can be fun, as some day centre patients show in these pictures.

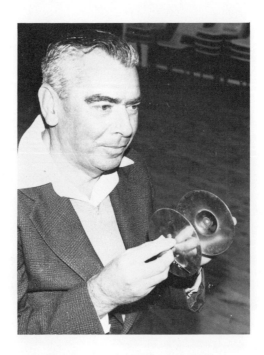

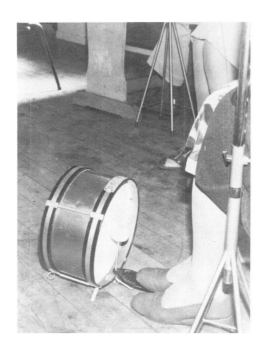

Instruments can be bought or improvised
— the foot pedal on a drum is helpful to a
disabled patient.

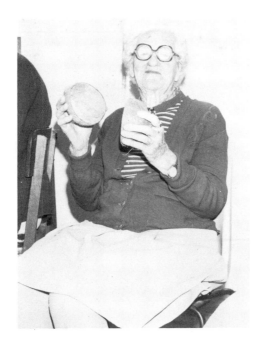

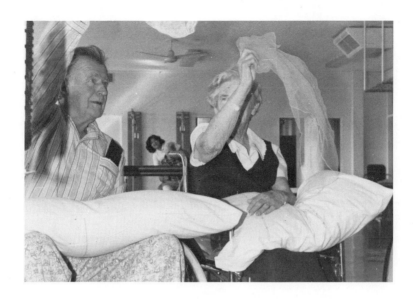

Scarves can be used for smooth movements and creativity, even some men find this enjoyable.

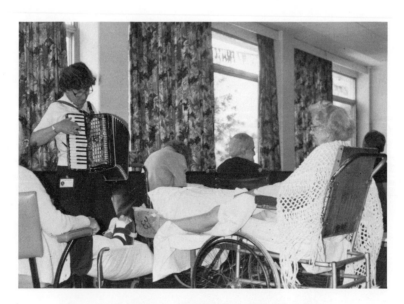

Even a minor toe "wiggle" is beneficial for the immobile patient, especially when the therapist can make a personal approach.

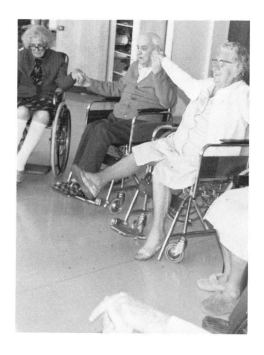

Holding hands in a circle gives a sense of "belonging".

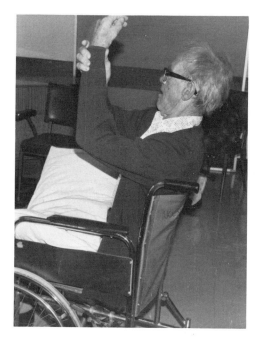

This patient has a left-sided (non-dominant hemisphere) stroke; he enjoys music for exercises and is using his "good" hand to raise the paralysed arm.

This patient has a visual field loss affecting his left eye, it was therefore essential to approach him from his "good" side.

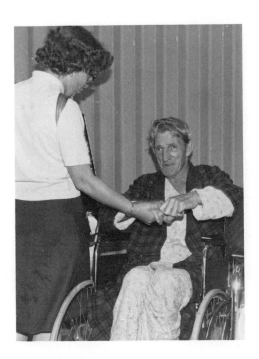

This patient has problems with rhythm of walking and with balance. He finds that music helps, but the physiotherapist walks nearby is case help is needed.

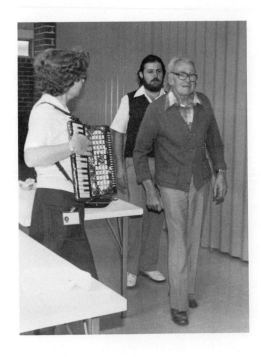

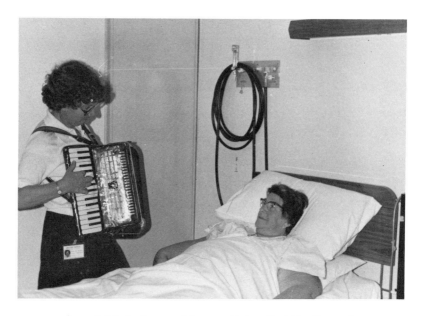

A portable instrument is essential so that the therapist
can work at the bedside.

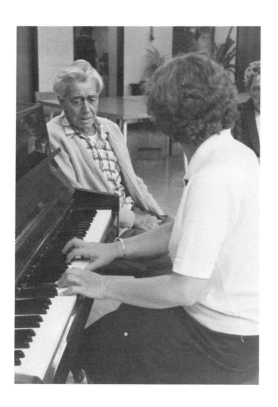

Music brings back memories for
many people.

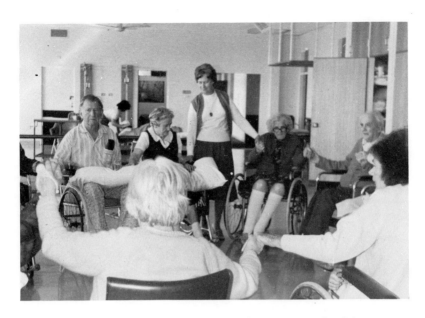

Relatives visiting the unit should be encouraged to join
in the activities — the gains will be great.

Don't worry if your sketches are
bad — it gives patients a pleasing
sense of superiority!

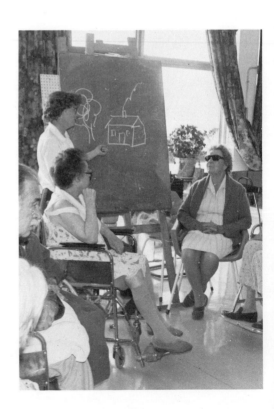

Fife, A.E. *Cowboy and Western Songs,* pub. Clarkson Potter, New York, U.S.A., 1969.

Keeping, C. (Ed.), *Cockney Ding-Dong,* pub. Kestrel, U.K., 1975.

Krone, M. *Music Sounds Afar,* pub. Follett, Chicago, U.S.A., 1958.

Large-Print Song Book, pub. Ulverscroft, Leicester, U.K., 1981.

Luboff, N and Stracke, E. (Editors), *Songs of Man,* pub. Prentice-Hall, New Jersey, U.S.A., 1968.

Sandbury, C. et al (Editors), *American Songbag,* pub. Harcourt, 1927.

Schaum, J. (Ed.), *Fifty Songs — Fifty States,* pub. Schaum Publications, Wisconsin, 1971.

CHAPTER 3: MUSIC IN REHABILITATION UNITS

In rehabilitation units there is generally little need for maintenance mobility work, since most people will be having physiotherapy as a routine part of their treatment programme. However from time to time there are people who are not included in individual physio, or who are having some specific problem, e.g. associated with balance or the rhythm of walking, and who will benefit from a combined approach by the two disciplines in a group setting. Work in this must be planned by the two therapists together to ensure maximum benefit to the patient — it may be decided that a slow waltz would be helpful in establishing walking rhythms, especially for a person with a lesion of the non-dominant hemisphere (which sometimes causes a loss or rhythmic sense and hence difficulties in walking, apart from those associated with general sensory loss and the loss of spatial awareness, which is so often a feature of strokes which affect the left side of the body). General sensory stimulation can also be provided through music, which helps those with sensory losses after brain damage — one can, for instance, place a tape recorder on the lap of a patient and place the flat of the hand against it to pick up maximum vibrations, to help re-build awareness of sensory in-put into the paralyzed hand and arm.

Patients who have a loss of visual fields or a lateral neglect as the result of stroke or trauma can be encouraged to use head-scanning movements in order to see the music therapist standing to one side of him, playing a portable instrument — this ties in well with Bobath techniques, which depend so much for their success on correct positioning of the head[1]. See also comments on page   re use of percussion instruments.

In general group work, the therapist must have a good idea of the diagnosis and treatment programme of each patient so as to be sure that the music therapy will reinforce whatever is being done by other disciplines and that it will fit in with the total approach to the patient. For example, one patient was suffering from anxiety about her bladder and continually asked to be taken to the toilet. It had been decided that she must be helped to build up her bladder capacity and to overcome as far as possible this anxiety, since continually going to the toilet made it impossible for her to take any sort of normal place in society. Therefore it was vital that her requests in music therapy group met with the same response as in other situations, otherwise the programme to modify her behaviour would fail. Similarly, if a patient is to be encouraged to sit up rather than collapsing to one side and asking to go to bed, then this must be dealt with consistently by all members of staff, including the music therapist. (Clearly such consistency is done for the benefit of the patient not with any punitive undertones!)

In some respects, a programme for a rehabilitation group is similar to that for a psychiatric group, but with some differences:—

(a) The level of participation is expected to be higher, so that patients are more aware of their surroundings, less out of touch with the outside world.

(b) Thus the type of quiz approach, although still appropriate, is presented in a more intellectual way generally, although even in a rehabilitation group there will be patients who have suffered severe cognitive deficit as the result of a stroke or other brain damage. Therefore the presentation must be geared carefully to each person's needs, as revealed in their case-history and by discussion with other staff.

There are difficulties when, in a group, there is a preponderance of people who are "on the ball" and a few who are very disabled intellectually. But by sensitivity to the attitude of each person one can use one's skills in personal relationships to make each person feel he is a valued member of the group. It is essential to be mobile for this. The therapist may choose to stand in the centre of the circle rather than on the outside, and, by placing oneself there, it is possible to get eye contact with each person in turn, even to the extent of sitting on the floor to play if a patient has difficulties with head posture. One of the things which wheel-chair people say they hate most is always having to look UP at people, and for this reason alone, the therapist must be ready to squat down or sit on the floor so as to reach eye level. (Try for yourself for just an hour or so sitting down when everyone else is standing up and talking to you — and you will gain a new understanding of the phrase, "talking down at people").

Many patients see the group music therapy session as recreation and fun (and perhaps some observers see it much the same way!), but there is underlying all that we do a therapeutic purpose, dove-tailing with work done by other therapists.

Sample Programme (to last about 45 minutes):

Use circle, 10-20 people at most, preferably 10-15.

1. Some people enjoy a welcome song, as described in section on psychogeriatrics. This technique has the advantage of helping people to learn each other's names, but some people find the handshake and the eye contact embarrassing, so do not make an issue of it!

If this is not done, you may like to start with some "name songs" which will introduce at least some of the people to each other, e.g. "Lily of Laguna," "Lilli" (from the film of that name, appeared 1952/3), "Mary's a grand old name," "Charlie is my darling," "Daisy," "A man called Peter," "Sally," and so on. Even though this will cover only a few names of people present, it gives the opportunity of talking about names, and may lead to revealing discussion of how people feel about being called by their first name — some older people find this humiliating and prefer Mrs........., but others find it merely friendly.

2. Suggest a waltz, e.g. "Skaters' Waltz," "Blue Danube," join hands around the circle. Use helpers to join up the circle if they are available, otherwise you may need to do some moving of wheelchairs to make sure that a right hemiplegic is not placed next to a left hemiplegic. Unless someone has a painful frozen shoulder, encourage some physical contact with paralyzed arm, at least get neighbour in the circle to touch the hand to give sensory stimulation. Move in time with the music, moving hands/arms and also if possible swaying whole body from side to side. (Good for circulation in buttocks, which become painfully sore from loss of circulation when one sits all day more or less immobile.)

3. Look around the circle for notable colour in clothing, suggest song to match and then ask who the song was for—e.g. "Alice Blue Gown" for someone in a blue dressing gown. The song need not mention clothes as such — any mention of colour will do, e.g. "White Christmas."

4. Main component of session may be chosen from a number of categories — a quiz such as was described on page   ; a particular composer, using recorded music as well as actual performance on piano or whatever is available, adding to this by giving a resume of his life and his place in general history, e.g. at Christmas or other major Christian festival, play excerpts from Handel's "Messiah" on tape, walking around with a small tape recorder so that everyone has a sense of belonging. Use pictures if large ones are obtainable to help to build up the sensory stimulation of the session as well as the enjoyment. One good idea is to use as the theme a place which people visit for holidays—e.g. for Australia, the Island of Bali; for U.K. one might choose Majorca or some part of Spain; in U.S.A. perhaps Hawaii would be appropriate. Some people in the posters, personal photographs — if reasonably clear — items holiday there, and this will add to the general conversation. Bring trave! posters, personal photographs — if reasonably clear! — items purchased there, artefacts of native origin, musical instruments, (e.g. a Balinese flute, with its — to our ears — unusual tuning), records of dances, etc. Vera Slabey, Director of Music Involvement at Mount Mathew, Wisconsin, has described such theme-related activities in a retirement community and nursing home, in which considerable time and effort can be spent on building up a large-scale programme of

music, costume, etc.[2] This will probably not be possible in the average hospital or nursing home, but by borrowing things from one's friends and gaining the co-operation of other staff, it is usually possible to build up a satisfying programme, which will provide intellectual stimulation, pleasant reminiscence, etc. The therapy behind such activity lies in the intellectual stimulation, the social contacts between patients, the opportunity for conversation generally, the sensory stimulation gained from listening to music, looking at pictures and other items, and general awareness of the world outside the hospital walls. It must be recognized that for some there will be an element of sadness, in that probably there will never again be an opportunity to go for a holiday to the place in question — although this is not necessarily so — and the discussion of the past always produces regrets for some. But this is a part of living; to insulate oneself against all sadness and all reminders of loss is as unhealthy as to dwell always on such loss, as some Victorians were said to do, having wax effigies made of the dead spouse, leaving rooms set up as if the dead person were still alive, and so on.

Always include a segment of the programme for free choice of music, so that all decisions are not made by the therapist; if someone has a strong wish for a song, try to get them to express the reasons for the choice, unless the person becomes too distressed by this. There is often a reason for a choice connected with personal life — ask about this, but not in a forceful way — leave the patient the opportunity for privacy.

For some there will be a need for private conversation afterwards, if the conversation has revealed an unresolved grief or resentment.

Be careful not to have the peak activity at the end, this leaves a "let-down" feeling when the session abruptly stops. Arrange the programme so that the elevation of mood is in the middle, with a gradual tailing-off towards the end. Close the session with a general activity — well-known song or some basic movement, e.g. clapping, so that there is a sense of unity at the end.

Links with Speech Pathology/Therapy:

In recent years there has been wide interest in the principles of melodic intonation therapy,[3] which makes use of the localization of music function, or of some of its aspects, in the minor hemisphere — the opposite hemisphere from that in which speech function is generally located.

It is inappropriate here to enter into detailed discussions of the mechanism underlying this therapeutic approach: the fundamental assumptions are:—

1. That there is extensive, even if not exclusive, representation of music function in the sub-dominant hemisphere.

2. That although speech is mainly represented in the dominant hemisphere, there are speech centres in the sub-dominant

hemisphere. Evidence for this lies in the fact that young children who have lost the dominant hemisphere in the neonatal period go on to develop normal speech even though they have in theory lost all the speech centres, and even with adults there are cases reported in the literature in which some speech has been regained following a hemispherectomy of the dominant hemisphere. Also the fact that aphasic patients can frequently sing the words of songs as well as the melody, and that emotive speech (expletives, etc.) is often retained despite asphasia caused by lesions of the dominant hemisphere, leads one to believe that there are speech centres, usually undeveloped, in the non-dominant hemisphere.

3. Thus in theory it should be possible to develop these centres even at an advanced age in order to gain some propositional speech (i.e. speech which enables the client to communicate, not merely mechanical speech of meaningless recitation).

4. In order to achieve such propositional speech, the client is taught musical phrases appropriate to the rhythm and intonation of normal speech, and thus gradually a vocabulary of useful phrases is built up. As the work progresses, the client is taught to change from singing to chanting (sing-song speech which is not unlike recitative of opera or oratorio), and from chanting to normal speech patterns.

When Sparks and Albert first put forward their theories and methods, there was discussion against allowing the client to sing songs he already knew. The present writer wrote protesting against such a relentless attitude, pointing out that the primary need of the aphasic is to relate with other people, and that to deprive him of one of the few modes of group activity still remaining to him was inhumane. Although no reply was received to this protest, it has been interesting to note that, in recent years, one no longer hears of edicts against social singing for the aphasic.

Difficulties arise when the music therapist is not present every day, since constant repetition is needed for this approach to have any hope of success. Before starting it is vital to assess the client's auditory discrimination—can he understand what is said to him, can he understand the meaning of any words he uses in his singing or is it merely mechanical, automatic speech? Unfortunately the answer to these questions is often "no" and then the idea of developing speech via music must be dropped, except for the pleasure afforded by social group activities involving singing, etc. But if it is apparent that the client does have good auditory discrimination, then one can embark on a programme of therapy, following the principles laid down by Sparks and Albert.

In order to test discrimination and understanding, the writer has used songs which include names of colours, and observed whether or not the client can pick out from a random collection of coloured slips the colour appropriate to the words of the song. e.g. When singing the words of

"White Christmas," can he pick out the white card? Similarly, when singing "Alice Blue Gown," can he pick out the blue card? The brown one when singing "Little Brown Jug," etc? Or, when singing "Daisy Bell" (a song which so many aphasic subjects delight to sing!), can he hold up two fingers to show that he understands what a bicycle built for two is? Or demonstrate by mime how one rides a bicycle to show that he knows what the song is about? And so on—each therapist will devise his own system of testing, depending on the cultural background of the client, using visual or auditory cues as required.

Once the musical phrases for communication have been evolved, it is of course essential that they are used consistently, and the client learns to relate the phrase which is used with an actual happening. e.g. If the phrase says "I need a cup of coffee," then the cup of coffee must be forthcoming, otherwise there is no gradual build-up of connection between the sound and its meaning. Similarly with what someone has said is the most important phrase for human dignity in the elderly aphasic, "I need to go to the toilet." Teaching this phrase must be so timed that the client is about to be taken to the toilet; one could imagine singing it as one progressed down the passage. The difficulty in this is that it can be seen just as funny, and given up for this reason. But if one can think rather of the problems of the patient in communication, of the helplessness of the person who cannot express his needs at all, the humour of the situation can be forgotten in the possible benefit which may be given to the client.

REFERENCES

1. Bobath, B. *Adult Hemiplegia, Evaluation and Treatment,* pub. Heinemann Medical, London, U.K., 1970.
2. Slabey, V. *Energy from our Elders — Music Involvement,* pub. by the author, Durand, Wisconsin, 1980.
3. Albert, M.L. & Sparks, R.W. & Helm, M.A. *Melodic Intonation Therapy for Aphasia,* Arch. Neurol., Vol. 29, August 1973, pp. 130-131.

CHAPTER 4: LOSS AND GRIEF IN THE AGED

In fact the only planning which one can do for work in loss and grief for the aged is preparatory study, so that one can respond appropriately to any situation which may arise. Each problem which one meets has its own special needs, which vary as much as individual people vary one from another. There are some things in common between all loss situations, and these one must learn from reading, from conversation with friends, acquaintances, relatives, strangers on long plane trips — in fact anyone who is willing to talk about loss and their reactions to it, thereby enlarging one's understanding of human need, and by giving their own personal experiences underlining the theoretical knowledge one has gleaned from one's reading. The author has vivid memories of a trans-Atlantic trip from Montreal to London in which most of the night was spent in discussing a personal problem of a neighbour in the plane, previously unknown, who was avoiding visiting a dying work-mate because he was frightened of what he might see and also uncertain as to how he would talk to his friend in the face of the certainty of death — whether he would be able to talk honestly or whether he would find he had to pretend. And in the face of fear and uncertainty, he did not go to the hospital at all. If you have a willing ear and a warm response, you will learn almost as much from such contacts as you will from textbooks.

Observations

(1) The Dying:

Elderly people do not on the whole appear to dread death as much as they dread incapacity and dependency; there seems to be a vast difference between one's response to a timely death, (i.e. one which is seen as coming at the end of a life which has been lived out to some degree of satisfaction, and one which occurs at an age when death is not surprising), and an untimely death — one which takes one by surprise and leaves one with a sense of disappointment at hopes left unfulfilled, years not lived and happiness not experienced. There are elderly people who fear death, or who at least fear the process of dying, with anxieties about pain, loneliness, loss of dignity and self-control, but generally it appears that the state of *being dead* is not a fearful one to the aged. Perhaps the thing one observes most frequently in those who do speak apprehensively of death is that they feel their lives have not been worthwhile, that — looking back over life — they see only the opportunities which have been missed, the failures rather than the successes. Sometimes this would seem to be part of a depressive response to illness and helplessness, and, if this is so, the music therapist has much to offer the dying person, in helping him to look back over life with a deeper sense of satisfaction than he has otherwise felt. (See below for suggestions as to how this may be achieved.) There are also some who dread the prospect of the after-life because they are burdened with a sense of guilt and thus believe that they are doomed to eternal life only in the form of eternal damnation. This is a particularly difficult problem for anyone to deal with; so much depends on one's own attitudes to life after death, to the creator as a loving or a vindictive God, to one's scale of values as to what constitutes a good or an evil life and so on. And even when one's own personal beliefs are taken into consideration, there is as well the ethical problem of how far one's own beliefs may be mentioned or presented to the dying patient if they are different from those of the patient, and in addition there are difficulties depending on whether one is working in a secular establishment or one which is sponsored by a religious organization of some kind. The author has always worked in organizations run by the State, in which religious teaching is frowned upon, although Chaplains are employed by the Department concerned, so that there is a recognition that spirtual well-being is a concern of the State.

Each therapist will have to solve this problem as he or she feels able, but often there is not such a difficulty as might be imagined, because people ask, "What do you think?" When this happens, it is fairly easy to present one's own personal views (acknowledging them to be personal), as long as they are not radically at odds with those views which the patient appears to hold. For instance, if someone is frightened of the judgment to come, which they believe will condemn them to damnation, but who then asks one's views, it is not difficult to offer comfort by saving, as the author has done, something to this effect — "I believe in a God who loves us and who is able to understand why we made the mistakes we did make. Just as parents can understand why their children get into muddles, and go on loving them just the same, so I believe that God loves us and forgives us when we are sorry for mistakes, and because he understands us, is not nearly as condemning about us as we are about ourselves." This is an intensely personal subject, but I know that we must not even think of working with the dying until we have worked out what we ourselves think about life and death, about death and life after death, about our own death in the future, and about any faith we may have or not have in a loving creator, supreme being, or whatever name we choose to use. With some people it is appropriate to suggest praying together, if this is compatible with our own beliefs — it can offer great comfort to the dying and to others who are in deep sorrow and anxiety, who have a genuine faith.

(2) The Bereaved:

Here reading is also helpful especially as there are some aspects of response to bereavement which people do not readily talk about, but which need to be ventilated. Professor Beverley Raphael, who holds the Chair of Psychiatry at the University of Newcastle, Australia, has found that in every bereavement there are moments (or in some instances strong feelings) of relief that the relationship has ended. Because such feelings are incompatible with the customary picture of grief, it is hard for the bereaved person to admit, even to himself, that he has a sense of freedom or relief in the death. The guilt which these feelings evoke, even if they are only momentary and transient, is great. Several writers have pointed out that the most difficult adjustments to death occur when the relationship has been an ambiguous one, because of the guilty feelings relating to the times of conflict, especially since the "normal" picture of grief accepted by the community is that of sadness unmixed by more complex emotions, and although local custom may lead the bereaved to be "brave" and hide this sorrow, we certainly do not expect any acknowledgment of feelings of release or freedom. Yet such feelings are common — how many of us have seen for example a widow, whom one had expected to be inconsolable and unable to stand on her own feet, take on a new lease of life in widowhood, leading the more perceptive to wonder whether her late husband's protectiveness was in fact a subtle form of repression — and similarly with some widowers, who make equally surprising adjustments to life alone. Unless one can adopt a realistic attitude to human relationships, one's counselling is likely to be ineffective and may even be destructive. If, for instance, a woman is becoming adjusted to life as a widow, and she has memories of her husband as difficult or demanding, her adjustment will be hindered by counselling which dwells only on the goodness/kindness, etc., of the deceased, since this will only lend extra weight to her guilty feelings at having herself found him difficult or unpleasant at times. We must give people the opportunity of saying openly, "He/she was sometimes a bit nasty," "Difficult to live with," "His untidiness drove me crazy and it is a relief to live at last in a tidy house," or any other such honest appraisal of the deceased. It is often necessary to give the bereaved a cue that such a feeling is all right to express; the precise wording of such a cue obviously depends on circumstances, the style of the counsellor, the personality of the bereaved, the extent of their disturbances and so on. But a comment such as this would rarely be found offensive: "I expect he had his moments of being hard to live with — all of us have! But sometimes when a person has died we feel we should pretend that they were perfect, and that can make us feel a bit guilty!" Because this statement admits that we *all* have faults, it permits the bereaved person to admit to the faults of the deceased without feeling guilty that he/she is behaving in an unnatural way. And from this it will become possible, if in fact the relationship has been a really difficult one, for the bereaved person to face honestly his/her own feelings of relief that the relationship is over, and make a far better adjustment to the death than if the pretence had been maintained that the deceased was a "plaster saint." Even a bereaved mother whose young child has died may have a guilty feeling of relief that at last she can get an unbroken night's sleep — and yet will feel intensely guilty at such an "unnatural" feeling, unless the counsellor gives her the cue that such a feeling is normal and natural.

The music therapist is not necessarily involved in all or any of these situations, but we all need to be thoroughly attuned to the complexities of grief and loss, so that we know how to give wise help to those in trouble, not treading the mindless path of conventional comfort and cheer, whether this is to bottle grief up, to speak only good of the dead, or any other of the common practices in speaking with those who are bereaved. People may need help to express their feelings of sadness, anger, etc., and the music therapist is in a good position to offer this help by playing appropriate music.

(3) Loss Situations:

In any acute hospital or long-term care facility, one meets people who have suffered loss other than bereavement; this may be the loss of body image and comeliness, as in a mastectomy, or colostomy, it may be loss of independence because of increased frailty or a stroke, amputation, arthritis or other condition. One meets also loss of self-esteem when physical problems have led to enforced retirement, inactivity, dependence on others and so on. In working with a wide cross-section of the population, the author has gained the impression that loss of independence is more feared than loss of life itself — people say, "I would rather be dead than have to depend on someone else to do everything for me." And one cannot help but believe that they mean what they say! For many, the loss of capacity to serve others is of paramount importance, people who have spent a lifetime doing things for others feel the loss of this keenly! It may be that for some there has always been a fragile self-esteem, which was maintained only by working for others — a potentially depressive personality — but for many even without being prone to depression, there is a strong sense of loss in having to be dependent on others. Nurses at one Sydney hospital recently completed a test period of dependency, in which trainee nurses spent a day (a) blindfolded, in order to have a deeper understanding of the needs of the visually impaired, and (b) being fed by a spoon by another person, to enter into the sense of humiliation felt by so many of those who have of necessity to be fed by a helper. The overall opinion was that being fed gave a sense of humiliation unequalled by any mimicry of disability in other areas. And yet this is a common occurrence, not only for those whose hand-function has been so reduced that being fed is essential, but also for those elderly persons who have become frail, slow or forgetful, for whom feeding is often a routine event in order to save time.

Some such people are no longer able to express their feelings of humiliation verbally but may do so (and here we need eyes to recognize the outburst of behaviour for what it truly is) by reverting to childhood incontinence, by anger and hostility or otherwise showing by non-verbal means their deep unhappiness and resentment. How can the music therapist help in such manifestations of loss and grief? Firstly it appears that to verbalise *for* someone is helpful: if we have feelings locked up inside us, it can give a sense of relief if someone else puts into words what we are afraid to express. We may fear that we shall be disapproved of or even punished for saying, for instance, how much we hate having food spooned into our mouths (often at a speed which is incompatible with real enjoyment of the food), but if someone else says, "It must be tiresome/miserable/awful (or whatever style of wording seems appropriate) to have to be fed," some at least of our anger and distress is alleviated and "defused" because we know that at last someone recognizes how we feel and cares enough about it to try to enter into our state of mind on the subject. And, as in so many other situations, the music therapist is in the position of being able to help people with their feelings because music therapy is not a matter of procedures, but of communication in an atmosphere of warmth and understanding in which unhappiness can be expressed without suspicion of grumbling and complaining.

When a patient clearly feels that his life has been a failure, that little or nothing has been achieved and that he might just as well have never lived, there is much the music therapist can do, if he/she truly believes that all human life is important and that even the humblest job has its role in society. By playing such a patient or client music which dates from his working life, one can help him to look back on his achievements with more satisfaction, supported by the therapist's own reassurance that his job was worthwhile. Some elderly women have been made to feel in recent years, (when women on the whole expect to have both family and career), that being a mother was not enough. One can use music to take them back to the past and to recall the difficulties under which many women had to work fifty years ago or so, without any of the modern equipment we take for granted today, perhaps battling against the problems of the depressions with their menfolk out of work on the dole*, having to cut down adult clothes for their children, inventing toys and games out of oddments, etc. All these achievements tend to be forgotten today, and this leads to the feeling that women who "only" brought up a family did not do enough. But music can take one back in a vivid way to that period of life, so that the achievements are seen in perspective as having a real value to society. Thus the self-esteem of the elderly is improved. Men too may need to have their

*The dole = unemployment relief money.

self-esteem bolstered by a clear recognition of the part they played in building today's world, a recognition of the difficulties which so many people faced between the wars, and in such therapy music is an ideal medium through which to work, because of the vivid memories which it evokes.

(4) Work with the Dying over a Lengthy Period

When terminal illness continues for any length of time, the work of the music therapist can have many and varied forms. For such work, recorded music can be used with good effects, both as a pleasant pastime, as an aid to pain relief, and, in a similar way to those methods already discussed, in counselling and in the verbalization of feelings.

Mount and Munro have written (in the Canadian Medical Journal)[1] of work in the Palliative Care unit in the Royal Victoria Hospital, Montreal, and the present author has little to add to the methods outlined in that article. Here the provision of equipment is of great importance: each patient must have his/her own tape-player and light-weight headphones, so that the music can be played at any time of day or night as the patient feels the need. This is vital — there are few opportunities for the dying to exercise power to make decisions, and this helplessness is in itself a source of distress and anger for many, so that to give the patient the chance to make his own decision as to whether or when the music is played is important. Also it enables music to be played in those dark lonely hours of the night or early morning when panic attacks of pain and fear so often occur. If the patient is extremely thin with hyper-sensitive skin, the headphones must be light enough, without undue clasping effects on the head, so that there is no discomfort in wearing them on the head. In extreme cases it may be necessary merely to place the headphones on the pillow next to the patient's ear so that the music can be heard without the headpiece being actually worn. Tapes can be built up of the patient's own selections of music to be heard, and the conversation which such choice entails gives to the therapist an excellent opportunity for discussion on more far-reaching topics than mere musical taste — why certain music is chosen, what significance it has for the person or in his relationships and so on. For times when someone is admitted outside the ordinary hours of the music therapist's work, there should be a good library of cassettes from which anyone can find something pleasant to listen to, until such time as more careful choice can be made. To have tape-player and tapes available immediately on admission does much to make the patient feel "at home" and to relieve some of the normal anxiety associated with being admitted to any hospital unit, and especially to a unit known to care for the dying. In this, the co-operation of nursing staff is essential, and clearly the nurses must have been helped to understand what the role of music therapy is in the care of the dying, so that their help is given readily.

Some people who have a period of weeks or even months in which they need to be in hospital, but are able to lead a life with some degree of activity, may enjoy playing instruments, making up their own songs, perhaps even songs which express their feelings about life and death or loss. A few will be able to write their own compositions out on paper, but for most it will be necessary for the therapist to write the music on paper from dictation, and probably also write a suitable accompaniment for pianoforte or guitar so that the songs thus composed can be given a hearing, and taped for permanence. A tape such as this will be a beloved bequest to some families.

It is by no means unknown for death to occur whilst the patient is listening to his chosen music, and — in the author's experience — nurses have observed that the patient has died with a smile on his face, despite extreme discomfort. The author is at present developing an idea in which the long-stay terminal patient is helped to record his life review, based on musical milestones, and this becomes a treasured possession which he can, if he wishes, bequeath to his family. For a great many people, there are milestones in life for which there are corresponding memories of music. Butler[2] has written of the value of the Life Review for the aged, as also has the present author[3], using music to enhance the reminiscence, and the recording of such review, combined with music, can be of great value as well as being a pleasant activity. Undoubtedly part of its value lies in the building of self-esteem and the giving of the therapist's undivided attention whilst the recording is being made (which can be spread out — and indeed will certainly need to be spread over several separate visits), and it may also give a sense of immortality because it is being recorded in permanent form. As has already been pointed out, the way in which the elderly reminisce about the past, (often the memories being evoked by music because of its emotional impact), should be regarded as a healthy activity rather than a pathological one. As we near the end of life, whether that life has been long or short, we need to look back and see our achievements or even our failures in some kind of perspective. Music is the ideal stimulus for reminiscence, and this fact is one of the strengths of music therapy in terminal illness at any age, and in geriatrics. For one younger terminal patient with whom the author is working on a continuing basis, (since his carcinoma is a slow-growing lesion), the milestones in music which feature on the tape are as follows:—

Early childhood —	Probably aged 3-4. Mother singing an Irish Lullaby. Being frightened on a rough ferry trip, and an itinerant musician singing the same lullaby, thereby reducing the young child's fear.
School —	First nursery songs, choir performance, being told to "mime" singing because of vocal quality — this was seen as a joke, not a disgrace!

	Dancing class, singing in the bus going to football games. Memories of specific funny music, mainly Stan Frieberg.
Courtship	First Rock and Roll music, going to see "Blackboard Jungle."
Early married life —	Particular songs of the period.
Wife's illness —	Listening to music as a shared experience.
Wife's funeral —	"Amazing Grace" played on bagpipes at the service.

The tape has been built up with music from various sources, and the patient's reminiscences are recorded between musical excerpts, or — in some instances — superimposed on the music, the volume of which has been reduced to allow the voice to come through. Two small tape recorders have been used at the bedside, so that music can be played simultaneously with the conversation. Jim is proud to be associated with what is probably a new use of music therapy in terminal illness and hopes that other therapists adopt the same idea; he says that he is amazed at how often music has been associated with important events in his life, and also speaks of the pleasure planning the recording has given him in between music therapy sessions. He has asked that the project should be described in print for the benefit of others, and is pleased at the idea of copying the tape as part of the author's clinical records. He hopes to leave the tape to his young daughters so that they may, in the years to come, have an idea of what kind of person he was, since they may only remember him as a person in bed.

So far the preparatory study which was mentioned in the opening paragraph of this chapter has been discussed only in terms of understanding the needs of the grieving, entering into the feelings of those who have suffered loss of body image, loss of acceptable appearance, loss of independence and self-determination. Important as this understanding is, the music therapist must also prepare for the musical demands made by such work; although one could sit down and say, "I have come to talk to you about your recent loss," the basic principle of using music therapy for the grieving is that music creates an atmosphere conducive to the open expression of feelings. And if this is to be achieved, then the therapist must be able to play spontaneously a very wide range of music, so that people's requests are filled on the spot — in the group, at the bedside or wherever else the therapist is in touch with the client. Obviously no one person can know every single tune ever written, but on must be willing to learn to play, upon a portable instrument such as guitar, accordion, flute or whatever, the songs and other pieces of music such as are frequently requested.

Repertoire

1. Learn songs which were popular in each decade — find old books of

music, from second-hand book shops, garage sales, Church fetes, ("White Elephant Stalls" as they are called in the British tradition!). Know at least one song from each year or two of this century, so that one can find something which was popular in the young adult life of any client living today. Check on the real date of first publications since many books of songs are published which give the year of the arrangement as if it were the date of first publication. e.g. The song usually attributed to Cat Stevens, "Morning has broken," is in fact taken from a folk melody of extreme antiquity, and uses words by an English poet, Eleanor Farjeon, which were published as a hymn in the book "Songs of Praise," first edition 1925! Similarly The Seekers' song, "The Carnival is over," was originally a Russian song, "Stenkarazin," and will be known as such to virtually every elderly Russian person. The Elvis Presley song, "It's now or never," will be known to every Italian person as "O Sole Mio," and so on; the list is endless.

2. Learn the tunes which were used for dancing at various times in this century; this is essential since songs of courtship are often requested by the grieving, and tunes which people dance to often become special to them ("our song") and it is these melodies which one needs to hear when grieving over the end of the relationship. Probably the melody played most often by the author in this situation is the Irving Berlin tune, "Always," followed closely by songs sung at wedding receptions, such as "Because," "I'll walk beside you," and so on.

3. Learn the main "hit tunes" from every year of the century so that, even if a client cannot think of a song or melody to ask for, one can offer an appropriate tune. Film music is a help in this — working onwards from "The Jazz Singer," featuring Al Jolson, through the 1930's, the 1940's, '50's, '60's, '70's up to the present day. (A good Encyclopedia Yearbook will provide entries for the release of films for each year, and from these lists it will be possible to find the music featured in each of these, whether it is a theme tune or a song or piece actually used in the story of the film or the musical show.) Such a list is undoubtedly daunting to the therapist who finds playing music difficult. Theoretically one can use records, but this destroys the immediacy of the situation — if a client is in deep distress, or has deep feelings which need ventilation, how much help can one give if one has to say, "I will try to get the tape and bring it tomorrow/next week or whatever?" The answer is obvious! Although the client will understand that one cannot play everything, it should be possible for the therapist to be able to play the second, third or even fourth request without undue loss of communication, especially if the therapist goes on to use this failure situation as a way in to communication with the client about his sense of failure in life. (This sense of failure is common in those who have suffered a disabling illness,

41

even though the client can recognize intellectually that such a feeling is unjustified.) When there is the prospect of a continuing relationship, one can of course find the music which was the first choice and bring it for a subsequent session, and build up a relationship through listening to music, talking about it and its significance in life. Most problems cannot be resolved in a single session, and although there is great need for spontaneity at that first encounter, with the therapist playing on the spot the music which has been requested, this does not lessen the value of the continuing therapy programme in which requested music can be found and played in later sessions. In fact the effort required to find some music enhances the patient's own self-esteem — the response is in effect thus: "I must be worth something if a busy person can go to all that trouble to find so-an-so for me." The finding of an obscure Australian Folk Song for an elderly man emphasized this — he repeatedly said, "Fancy going to all that trouble for ME!" (He had grown up on the goldfields and recalled the miners singing a song called "Take me back to Bendigo"; a search at the public library located a book which contained the song, a copy was made for the patient and for the therapist, in case of future need, and some details noted as to the source of the song.)

Advice to the therapist involved through music in grief counselling would be — Be Knowledgeable and Be Brave — better to have a poor performance of a tune than not to try at all! As a last resort, ask the client to sing it to you so that you can learn it — the therapeutic spin-off of this is considerable, but unfortunately few clients are brave enough themselves to do it.

In all therapeutic work, it is essential to work as a member of a team; one must not work alone but with co-operation and communication with others. People do produce results sometimes working as a "one-man band" but the long-term effects in the establishment as a whole are likely to be destructive because other team members will cease to give referrals or will in more subtle ways withdraw support from the errant therapist. Information gleaned in discussion with patients must be passed on, so that work with the client will have a unity of approach, with shared information to assist that approach. Obviously some clients relate better to one therapist and some to another, but this is common in any therapeutic work and can be accepted by the team. What is destructive to teamwork is the attitude "So-and-so only works for me," or "I am the only one who understands so-and-so." All therapists or would-be therapists should read the writings of Safilios-Rothschild on this topic, and learn to be aware of their own behaviour and possible motivation for wanting to play a lone hand. Accept the responsibility and the restrictions but also the benefits of working in a team if you want to bring the utmost good to the client. These may seem harsh comments or warnings, but the music therapist is especially at risk either of actually working in isolation, of being suspected of working in isolation or of having isolation thrust upon him by circumstances. We are usually not trained in a paramedical establishment, and thus are not accustomed, as are physical, occupational or speech therapists to working in a clinical setting, and it is thus all too easy to find oneself alone. In some hospitals or clinics even the best endeavours of the music therapist will not achieve teamwork, but one must continue to try, albeit without denying one's own role in the care of patients. The surgeon, the social worker, the nurse — all must have some comprehension of music as therapy for the dying patient, the bereaved and the grieving, so that referrals are appropriate or — if a policy is adopted which enables the music therapist to see all patients in a particular unit for assessment and programme planning where this is likely to be helpful — to ensure that adequate time is allowed for the individual therapy as required. One anecdote of an incident in 1981 at a hospital in which the author works will illustrate this. A fairly intense conversation was in progress with a patient when the trolley arrived to take the patient to X-ray.

R.B.:   "Oh John, does she have to go right away!"

Charge Nurse: "No, how long do you need to finish off — will ten minutes be O.K.?"

R.B.:   "Yes, thanks — that should be about right."

Exit wardsman, nurse and trolley to wait outside in the corridor. Later, after patient gone to X-ray:

Charge Nurse: "Ruth, if ever you are in the middle of an important discussion with someone, don't ASK us if you can finish off — just TELL US!!"

(It will be recognized from the foregoing conversation, which is reported verbatim, that the hospital is an unusual one in that friendly relations exist between all levels of staff so that excellent communication is maintained between doctors, nurses, therapists, domestic staff and so on. It has only suggested that such communication improves patient care because it helps junior staff who may notice a change in a patient's condition or some feature of an illness which has not been noticed by more senior staff to express their anxiety, give details of what has been observed and so on. In an intensely hierarchical structure such ease of communication may not be achieved, and patient care can suffer if junior staff are unwilling to speak their views.)

Although these remarks are written in the context of terminal care, they are equally true of any therapeutic situation, in any hospital or in special school. Teamwork is the only way to achieve optimum levels of client care and the music therapist must be willing to learn how to work in this manner.

REFERENCES

1. Munro, S. & Mount, B. *Music Therapy in Palliative Care,* Can. Med. Assoc. Jnl., Vol. 119, No. 9, November 4th, 1978.
2. Butler, R.N. *Successful Aging and the Role of the Life Review,* Jnl. Amer. Geriatrics Soc., Vol. XXII, No. 12, pp. 529-534, December, 1974.
3. Bright, Ruth, *Music in Geriatric Care,* p. 5 onwards, pub. (re-issue) Musicgraphics, Lynbrook New York, 1980.

RECOMMENDED READING

Bright, Ruth. *Music and the Management of Grief Reactions,* in Nursing and the Aged, ed. Burnside, I.M., pub. McGraw-Hill, 1981, p. 137ff.

Hinton, J. *Dying,* pub. Penguin Books, Harmondsworth, U.K., 1967.

Kubler-Ross, E. *On Death and Dying,* pub. Tavistock, London, U.K., 1970.

Parkes, C.M. *Bereavement: studies in adult grief,* pub. Tavistock, London, U.K., 1972. Penguin paperback, 1975.

Safilios-Rothschild, C. *The Sociology and Social Psychology of Disability and Rehabilitation,* pub. Random House, New York, U.S.A., 1970. Especially section on team-work.

RESOURCE MATERIAL

16mm Film, *The Last Days of Living,* Canadian Film Board, (filmed in the Palliative Care Unit, Royal Victoria Hospital, Montreal), shows some music therapy.

CHAPTER 5: CREATIVITY IN MUSIC THERAPY FOR THE AGED

It would be wrong to assume that the elderly only like music which is familiar; this may be true for some, and perhaps even for a large proportion, but it is certainly not a universal truth. Many elderly people enjoy "Pop" music, keeping well in touch with modern trends, although with more selective approach than many of the young, who so often appear to need to follow slavishly the popularity charts, without much reference to their private likes and dislikes. It must be recognized that in any geriatric hospital or nursing home, any club or day centre for frail aged or for well aged people, there may be a vast span of years between oldest and youngest. For instance, because of the nature of their disabilities, one meets in a geriatric unit people in their twenties who have suffered brain damage in car accidents, people in their thirties who are far advanced with multiple sclerosis, people in their forties who have had space-occupying lesions in the cortex or who have had strokes, people in their fifties who have had strokes or incapacitating rheumatoid arthritis and so on. (It is worth noting that in the state of Western Australia, thanks to the teaching and influence of Professor Dick Lefroy, the term "Geriatric" is no longer used, and units which are labelled thus elsewhere are referred to as Extended Care units; because of the nature of the care and treatment they are able to give, they cater for far more than the elderly population who are in need of care, and provide extended care for M.S. patients, motor vehicle accident cases and others who are still in their early or middle adult years.)

People in early or middle years will not enjoy an exclusive diet of the songs of the pre-war period — and this is also true of any group of people, even of advanced age. One must provide variety, and music group activities can help to keep people in touch with today's world by introducing them to music of today, selected with care and played in a manner less noisy than the average Disco, or whatever term is fashionable for places frequented by the young and playing extremely loud music. Learning new things is in itself a creative experience, since one's horizons are extended, one's opinions challenged and one is led into new ways of thinking or listening. Thus a programme of music therapy, wherever it is taking place, should include some up-to-date music to stimulate thought and conversation (not to mention argument, in many instances!) At the time of writing, Bette Midler's song, "The Rose", is popular with all ages.

Some people enjoy playing tuned and untuned percussion instruments: it is unfortunately true that some feel it to be childish, perhaps it is those who fear the deterioration of old age who react in this way, or it may be the mode of presentation which is at fault. But many older people do enjoy orchestra/band work, especially if it is made a fairly demanding activity, not a mindless banging out of an unchanging beat.

Instrumental work can be introduced by appropriate records or films which show the percussion section of an orchestra, or by attendance at a concert in which percussion music will be included. Instruments should be chosen for their tonal quality — beware of kindly donors who fob off tinny instruments which produce a feeble tinkle or a dull clunk. Spend as much money as you can to get good quality things.

Creativity can be encouraged by asking the group or the individual to work out a routine of instrumental work to suit the music which has been selected and, as an adjunct to this, choosing what type of music the group will use in the first place. The group may enjoy improvising, i.e. playing the instruments in an unplanned way, having what are in effect conversations on the instruments. However before deciding on such an activity, be sure that the group —

(a) can hear what is going on,

(b) knows each other fairly well,

(c) feels happy at doing this.

Unless people feel at home with one another they will be overcome with shyness and the activity will be a minor disaster. Also if anyone in the group is impaired of hearing, the activity will not be enjoyed. Some people are frightened of an unstructured activity and prefer to have their playing planned for them, perhaps even set out on charts. Many elderly people are apprehensive about their ability to learn something new — not, it must be pointed out, because they are actually incompetent, but because society has for so long said "You can't teach an old dog new tricks" that the old have come to believe it. And of course amongst the frail and forgetful, there are indeed some to whom one cannot teach new skills, who will be more relaxed with a simple planned structure — we must be careful not to make the music session one more failure experience, to add to the many that people have already experienced.

Bells which are made in a set are helpful in instrumental work: each person has a bell which is coloured according to its pitch, so that if one has several sets, one knows that all red bells produce the same note and so on. They are also numbered on the ends, for those who prefer to work by number. Charts can then be drawn which give tunes in terms of numbers or colours. In the first instance, and perhaps always, it will be necessary to have a conductor who points to each person or group of players in turn.

The group will gradually acquire not only the skill of playing when the right moment arrives, but also — more difficult? — the skill of stopping at the right moment! Although not all tunes can be contained within the single octave, there are many which are written thus and there is the possibility of group composition to create new tunes to play on the bell set.

Chime bars, especially those in which the bars can be detached if necessary, can be used effectively. Or one may prefer to have individual chime bars in which each person has his own, and charts similar to the bell charts can be used, with the difference that a greater range of melodies can be attempted if one buys chime bars which cover more than the octave. This demands more concentration because of the need to differentiate between C and C', or between F and F#, but given the right group more ambitious work can be attempted. Sets of chime bars can be used to help those with a one-sided neglect to cross the midline. (In certain forms of brain damage, there is a neglect of one side of the body, and the patient finds it hard to look across the midline of the body, or to move the arm across to the opposite side. Musical instruments which "force" the player to make such movements are helpful in therapy.)

Using chiffon scarves can be pleasant: it provides for creativity in the movements which are performed with the scarves. Mimicry, in which one person tries to mirror the movements done by another, is demanding but fun. And of course all these activities can be planned with an underlying therapeutic intent, to encourage certain arm movements, range of shoulder movements, and so on. Music for this should be imaginative in itself — Grieg's "Morning," with its changing moods, is one example of evocative composition which assists creativity in movement; in fact all the Peer Gynt suite is helpful.

Most music therapy activities provide an experience of success and not (as with so many other life situations for the sick aged) of failure. People look forward to music therapy sessions, whether these are in an in-patient facility for rehabilitation, long-stay care in nursing home or sheltered accommodation such as a frail aged hostel, a day ward for out-patient treatment, or a social day centre based on a hospital or in a club atmosphere. It is this quality of pleasurable anticipation which is the greatest strength of music therapy, and it affects the whole life-style. An occupational therapist describes how a patient dresses herself much more competently on music mornings than on other days because she wants to be sure of getting to the music therapy session in time. A physiotherapist describes how a patient with severe problems in walking gets going more easily because he wants to get to the music therapy session right at the beginning. A withdrawn and electively mute patient sits up straight and sings audibly some of the songs which are chosen, eventually choosing a song for himself. A man with a severe depression, and almost mute, talks firmly of film music from his youth and becomes known as the ward's Film Expert, thereby gaining a defined role in the ward population, extending his social contacts and his status by his expert knowledge. All these things are the substance of music therapy, and — by careful observation rather than numerical charting systems — the effects of music therapy can be proved. One can observe how much more social interaction there is after a music session than at the corresponding time on other days, other members of staff can note how much more communicative their patients are after a music session — for example, a social worker in one area of the hospital always chooses the time immediately after music therapy to approach patients because she finds that they are more accessible to conversation then, compared with other times. This is not to say that music therapy always makes us smile or laugh, it is not entertainment except at a superficial level. But even if the music leads to tears, it is still of value when those tears can be "used" for the benefit of the patient.

It is true that for many psychogeriatric patients one has to start each day a-fresh, introducing oneself anew each session, reminding people each session of what the day of the week is when music therapy happens. But even if this continues indefinitely, is the session any the less valuable for that reason, so long as it brings even temporarily a sense of pleasure and self-esteem and a capacity to relate to others in a group?

A quotation from Burnside's book, "Nursing and the Aged", on page 220, sums it all up thus:

> "Just because a message may never be received does not mean it is not worth sending."(Segaki, translated by David Stockton).

Just because our clients may forget for week after week, month after month and possibly year after year until eventually they remember who we are, why we are there and even what day of the week it is that music happens, does not mean that it is not worth doing.

In investigating the value of music therapy, we must beware of what Professor John Hinton, of the University of London, referred to as "Scientism";[1] whilst it is unfortunately true that some people, including decision-makers who determine the staffing of hospitals and special schools, demand statistics and numbers, we must never lose sight of the fact that music is concerned with the emotions and not the pulse rate, with self-esteem and not with posture, with communication and not handwriting. All of these concrete, measurable items may be an indication of how our therapy is progressing, but they are not the stuff of which therapy is made. Of all the therapies, music speaks to the heart of mankind and not to statistics.

REFERENCES

1. Hinton, J. Private communication.

SUMMING UP

In all the aspects of music therapy which have been discussed, there is no discussion of research, of verification of data by controlled experiments. To some therapists this may cast doubts upon the use of music in therapy for the aged — for some people, Chi square tests and crossover double blind tests are the only source of reliable information! But how much use are they in the field of geriatrics? How can we get two truly matched samples of subjects, one group of whom will receive music therapy whilst the others do not? We need to consider the realities of geriatric care before attempting such statistical analysis. Clearly there are some topics which lend themselves to investigation in a controlled way: a project undertaken by the author in 1975 demonstrated this[1]. The experiment was designed to find out how much similarity there is in people's perception of the mood of music. (It is necessary to know this when attempting work in clinical improvisation, since there is no point in the therapist playing music which *she* perceives as angry, in an attempt to help externalize hidden hostility in the client, if the client perceives the music as peaceful and restful!) In this study it was found on statistical analysis that there was general agreement on the mood perceived in the music, but also some bizarre "misinterpretations" of mood, mainly from those with grave psychiatric illness. The groups consisted of 60 patients in a psychiatric hospital, in a geriatric rehabilitation and long-stay hospital with some general wards, and 60 control subjects. Whilst this was of interest and of value, there are many aspects of music therapy for the aged which cannot be tested with any expectation of meaningful results. For example in reality orientation with institutionalized patients, there are many variables to be considered: —

How long have the subjects been in hospital?

To what extent do they have memory loss?

Is it long-term memory loss or only for recent events?

What was their interest in music before entering the institution?

What is their presenting diagnosis?

What other pathology do they exhibit?

What was their life experience in their pre-morbid life?

What was their pre-morbid pattern of social relationships?

Do they have language problems as the result of migration?

Have they lost a measure of communication because of stroke resulting in aphasia?

Do they suffer from confabulation?

Do they show word-salad in their speech?

Is their hearing impaired?

Is their vision impaired?

Have they retained any social support from "the outside", which might alter their memory for events, and awareness of the outside world?

From this list it will be seen that to assemble two identical groups of subjects for research, with identical physical, social, emotional and psychological status, with the same length of institutionalization, the same degreee of social support from family, the same diagnosis, the same pre-morbid life style and musical experience, is, one can safely say, impossible. Yet performance in psychological tests, including those which involve music, is profoundly affected by all these factors and probably others which have not been listed. And the same is true of many other aspects of music therapy which, one might imagine, would lend themselves to investigation.

Probably the most important aspect of music therapy is the happiness which it brings; it provides our elderly clients with a "success situation" rather than an experience of failure, it emphasizes in almost every programme the things which the disabled or frail elderly can do, rather than those which they cannot. In those few situations, such as helping a client to ventilate an obstructed grief, in which the aim is apparently a negative one, the ultimate effects, in terms of increased inner peace, amply justify the temporary expression of sadness which is entailed.

One may sum up the value of music therapy for the aged by saying that it speaks to the heart and the spirit: to achieve the best results, one must plan ahead with sensitivity to the needs of each group and each individual, and then work in a spirit of hopefulness and empathy so that there may be a real benefit of some kind to each of our clients.

REFERENCE

1. Bright, Ruth. *Perception of Mood in Music,* A statistical comparison of two patient populations and a control group. pub. Proceedings of 2nd National Conference, Australian Music Therapy Association, Melbourne, Australia, 1976, pp.95-104.

INDEX

Achievement, 2

Adaptation, loss of in aged, 5

Aggression, 22, 23

Alzheimer's Disease, 17

Amputation, 9, 36

Anger, 22

Anxiety, 8, 9, 15, 27

Aphasia, 30ff

Arteriosclerosis, 17

Arthritis, 36

Auditory Discrimination, 31

Bereavement, 35ff

Bladder training, 27, 28
  see also incontinence

Bobath methods, 26

Brain damage, 2, 17, 27
  see also car accident, stroke

Cancer, 2
  see also death, dying, pain

Car accident, 2, 45
  see also motor vehicle accident

Cerebrovascular accident
  see stroke

Choice, 20, 22, 30

Clinical team
  see teamwork

Cognitive deficit, 28
  see also dementia

Communications, 2, 22,48

Counselling by M.T., 5, 36, 37, 38, 42

Creativity, 45ff

Custodial care, 3

C.V.A.
  see stroke

Deafness, 46

Death, dying, 33ff

Decision-making, 20, 30, 38

Dementia, 4, 19, 23, 24
  see also pseudodementia

Dependency, 36ff

Depression, 18, 36, 47

Discharge from hospital, 16

Disinhibition, 16, 17

Disorientation, 4

Disseminated sclerosis
  see multiple sclerosis

Emotional difficulties, 10, 15
  see also anxiety, fear, etc.

Empathy, 50

Ethnic
  see migrant

Exercises, 7ff, 10, 11, 14

Extended care, 45

Eye contact, 28

Failure, 19, 34, 37, 41, 46, 47

Fear, 9, 38

Femur, fractured, 8

Folk Music, 24ff

Grief, 4, 30, 33ff, 50

Group work, 10, 18ff, 28

Health, general, of aged, 3ff, 7

Hemiplegia
  see stroke

Hemisphere (dominant, non-dominant), 30, 31

Hospitals, 3, 7, 16, 30

Hospital staff, 20
  see also teamwork

Hostels, 16

Huntington's Disease, 17

Immigrants
  see migrant

Improvisation, 1, 2, 49

Incontinence, 4, 12, 16

Independence, 3

Individual therapy, 8

Instruments,
  see percussion

Intellectually handicapped, 17
Intellectual stimulation, 30

Korsakow's syndrome, 17

Liability, 18
Learning, 46ff
Life Review, 25, 39ff
    see also reminiscence
Loss, 4, 34ff, 36ff
    see also Bereavement
        Death
        grief
Love, the need to give, 19

Maintenance therapy, 10
    see also exercises, mobilization
Marriage difficulties, 9
Melodic Intonation Therapy, 30ff
Memory loss, 17, 22
Migrants, music for, 15
    see also folk music
Mobilization, mobility, 4, 8, 14, 22
Motivation, 15, 47
Motor vehicle accident, 17
    see also car accident
Movement with music, 47
    see also exercises
Multiple sclerosis, 18, 45
Music therapy, definition, 1ff

Neglect, lateral, 31, 56
Nursing homes, 3, 10, 16, 17, 30

Orthopedic patients, 8

Pain, 8, 38
Palliative care, use of music therapy,
    38ff
Parkinson's Disease, 17
Percussion instruments, 39, 46ff
Physical therapy (physiotherapy), 7, 14,
    27
    see also exercises
Pictures, drawing for group work, 20,
    21

Post-operative care, 8, 14
Privacy, required, 30
Pseudodementia, diagnosis of, 5
Psychiatric hospitals, 10, 16ff
Psychiatric illness, 10, 16ff
Psychiatric patients, 2, 10, 16ff
Psychological needs, 15
Psychotherapy, 1

Quiz, in group work, 21, 22, 28

Reality orientation, 49
Reassurance, required, 9
    see also counselling
Recorded music, 7, 9, 22, 29, 38ff
Recreation, 3
Rehabilitation, 21, 27
Relationships, 1, 2, 24, 28
Relaxation, 1
Religious beliefs, 34ff
Reminiscence, 2, 19, 25, 30
    see also Life Review
Re-orientation, 21, 49
Repertoire, of therapist, 40ff
Research, 49, 50
Retarded
    see intellectually handicapped

Schizophrenia, 17
Self-esteem, 36, 42, 48
Sensory losses, stimulation, 20, 27, 30
Sexual problems, 9
Singalongs, 1, 2, 22
Songbook, 22, 24, 26
Spasticity, 9
Speech therapy, 30ff
Spinal injury, 9
Stroke, 7, 9, 10, 16, 36
Success, sense of/experience of, 27f, 50

Taped music, 57, 61
    see recorded music
Tape recorder, player, 27, 38

Taste in music, 45
   see also choice, decision-making
Teamwork, 1, 3, 7, 8, 9, 18, 27ff, 42ff
Traction, 8

Wandering demented patient, 24
Women, role of in society, 37
Wheelchair, 10, 28
   see also exercise programme